Management of Macular Hemorrhage

Lars-Olof Hattenbach
Editor

Management of Macular Hemorrhage

Springer

Editor
Lars-Olof Hattenbach
Augenklinik des Klinikums Ludwigshafen
Ludwigshafen
Germany

ISBN 978-3-319-65875-9 ISBN 978-3-319-65877-3 (eBook)
https://doi.org/10.1007/978-3-319-65877-3

Library of Congress Control Number: 2018936521

Printed on acid-free paper

This Springer imprint is published by the registered company Springer International Publishing AG part of Springer Nature.
The registered company address is: Gewerbestrasse 11, 6330 Cham, Switzerland

Preface

Retinal hemorrhage involving the macula is a typical complication in a variety of ocular disorders including age-related macular degeneration, arterial macroaneurysm, valsalva retinopathy, or trauma. To date, the ideal approach to the management of macular hemorrhages remains controversial. However, given the different types of hemorrhage classified as subretinal, intraretinal, pre-retinal, or vitreous and its varying impact on visual function, it is likely that multiple treatment approaches are needed.

This book provides insights and understandings into the complexities of macular hemorrhage and gives a systematic overview of therapeutic approaches that cover the most important situations a vitreoretinal surgeon might encounter when treating patients with this disorder.

In the initial chapters, we describe the pathophysiology and the clinical course of the various types of macular hemorrhage and provide a clinically useful, evidence-based classification that enables ophthalmologists to make an accurate diagnosis, give a more reliable prognosis, and identify those patients eligible for treatment.

Lastly, this book summarizes the various approaches ranging from minimally invasive to complex vitreoretinal surgery, thereby allowing to select tailored treatments that can greatly improve the chances of improving vision in each individual case. Experienced vitreoretinal surgeons describe their surgical techniques, personal observations, and preferences how to approach treatment, orienting therapy toward the different types of macular hemorrhage.

Supplemented by case presentations, clinical photographs, and an extensive review of the literature, this book contains all relevant information a vitreoretinal surgeon needs to know about clinical decision-making, typical pitfalls or surgical techniques and strategies such as subretinal drainage, macular translocation, autologous RPE-choroidal transplantation, or the combined use of fibrinolytic and anti-VEGF agents, and invites the reader to explore the advantages and disadvantages of various approaches to the management of macular hemorrhage.

Ludwigshafen, Germany — Lars-Olof Hattenbach

Contents

About the Author

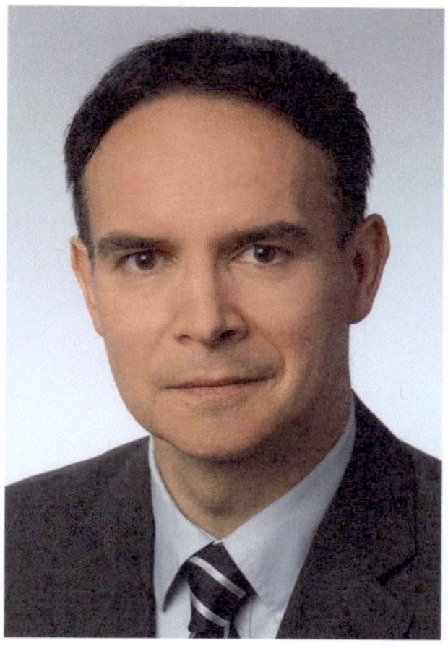

Lars-Olof Hattenbach, M.D., F.E.B.O. is a professor of ophthalmology and chairman of the Department of Ophthalmology at Ludwigshafen Hospital, Germany. After ophthalmology and internal medicine residency training at the Johannes Gutenberg University Mainz and the Charité Berlin, he completed his ophthalmology residency and a subspecialty training in vitreoretinal surgery at Goethe University Frankfurt, where he received his primary degree and served as a consultant and lecturer. Professor Hattenbach maintains an active research and teaching profile and has been the principal investigator in numerous clinical trials encompassing diseases of the posterior segment. He is a reviewer or associate editor for multiple international journals, authored books and chapters on the treatment of retinal diseases and has published extensively in the field, with more than 90 articles to his name in peer-reviewed journals.

The Pathophysiology of Subretinal Hemorrhage

1

Salvatore Grisanti and Swaantje Grisanti

Introduction

Subretinal hemorrhage (SRH) may be associated with a variety of diseases as described in various chapters of this book. The natural course of SRH often leads to significant and permanent visual impairment, predominantly in cases when the macula is affected. Although there are a substantial number of publications related to clinical appearance and outcome, the knowledge about the pathophysiology is limited. In a histopathologic study on 176 human eyes with age-related macular degeneration, Green and Key [1] found that SRH was associated with loss of photoreceptors and thinning of the outer nuclear layer, but sparing of the inner nuclear layer. Disciform scars were associated with this same pattern of loss of the first retinal neuron and sparing of the second retinal neuron.

With the development of vitrectomy in the 1970s, the interest in understanding the chronology and effects of SRH grew due to the potential of becoming removable. The first experimental studies were performed in a rat model. Koshibu described in three consecutive publications [2–4] that erythrocytes in the subretinal space were engulfed by macrophages that underwent degeneration and were phagocytized by retinal pigment epithelial cells and by Mueller cells. The SRH was resorbed in 21–60 days, after which yellow-brown deposits could be seen by ophthalmoscopy. Koshibu observed that the retina overlying the hemorrhage became intensely degenerated over a period of months. He attributed this retinal degeneration to iron toxicity. This assumption was based on previous studies analyzing the direct effect of ferrous and ferric or metallic iron on the retina [5–8].

In 1982 Glatt and Machemer [9] performed similar experiments in a rabbit and a cat model. The authors injected fresh autologous blood into the subretinal space and studied the hemorrhages both clinically and histologically. They found that **one hour** after injection, the subretinal space contained erythrocytes, leukocytes, and occasional thin fibrin strands. Retinal changes were minimal and limited to occasional photoreceptor edema. The outer nuclear layer showed no pyknosis or karyolysis, and the inner retina was normal. At **one day**, however, there was marked damage of the photoreceptor cells characterized by edema and disintegration of the photoreceptors and pyknosis of the outer nuclear layer. Some photoreceptors had been pulled off the retina by contraction or movement of the blood clot, or both. The changes were more marked in non-vascularized parts of the retina and in areas with high detachments than in areas with low detachments. After **three days** fibrin was present in the subretinal space. Occasional macrophages

S. Grisanti, M.D. (✉) · S. Grisanti, M.D.
Department of Ophthalmology,
University of Luebeck, Lübeck, Germany
e-mail: salvatore.grisanti@uk-sh.de

L.-O. Hattenbach (ed.), *Management of Macular Hemorrhage*,
https://doi.org/10.1007/978-3-319-65877-3_1

containing red cell fragments had become evident in the subretinal space. The inner retina exhibited the degenerative changes already noted at day 1: cystoid spaces and pyknosis. Additionally, thinning of the outer nuclear layer, indicating the onset of karyolysis, was noted. By **seven days**, the photoreceptor cells were almost absent and the retinal damage severe. The outer nuclear layer had undergone severe karyolysis. The appearance of the inner nuclear layer ranged from normal to severe karyolysis, and cystoid space formation with more abnormalities in areas of non-vascularized retina was observed. At **two weeks**, most of the subretinal clot had disappeared. No fibrin and only a few erythrocytes were evident in the subretinal space. Many macrophages were found in the subretinal space and in the retina. The outer nuclear layer was completely absent. The inner nuclear layer showed various changes, ranging from normal to little change, which was seen in the following 2 weeks. All subretinal blood had been resorbed by **four weeks**.

SRH in rabbits led to irreversible retinal destruction within 1 day. The authors concluded that the mechanism of the destruction of the overlying retina consists of a combination of a diffusion barrier by the clot, mechanical damage to the outer segments by contraction of the clot, and iron toxicity.

It took almost a decade before a further related study was published in 1991 [10]. Toth et al. [11] observed an initial clot organization with retraction of fibrin strands in a cat model. In clots more than 1 h old, fibrin was associated with tearing of sheets of photoreceptor inner and outer segments. Later, degeneration progressed to involve all retinal layers overlying the most dense areas of fibrin in the clots. Hemorrhages into subretinal blebs containing tissue plasminogen activator did not form fibrin strands or cause photoreceptor tearing. These findings highlighted the potential for improved retinal survival if organized subretinal clots can be eliminated soon after formation. Subsequently, the authors described as early as 1992 the facilitated clot lysis followed by removal of subretinal hemorrhage when using recombinant tissue plasminogen activator.

Bhisitkul et al. used a rabbit model of autologous SRH to determine the morphologic features and time course of retinal damage, characterize the apoptotic mechanisms of photoreceptor cell death, and assess the role of iron toxicity and macrophage activity in blood-mediated cell death [12]. They disclosed that photoreceptor degeneration initiated 48 h after exposure to subretinal blood and progressed over 7 days. They correlated the presence of iron in the photoreceptor layer with photoreceptor degeneration and concluded that photoreceptor toxicity occurs at least in part by apoptosis and is associated with iron migration to the photoreceptor layer.

More recently Notomi et al. [13] demonstrated that SRH accompanies a significant increase in extracellular ATP and that extracellular ATP initiates a neurodegenerative processes through specific ligation of purinergic receptor P2X and ligand-gated ion channel, 7 (P2RX7; P2X7 receptor). This assumption was based on increased extracellular ATP levels in the vitreous samples of AMD patients with subretinal hemorrhage compared to control vitreous samples. Additionally, extravascular blood induced a massive release of ATP and photoreceptor cell apoptosis in co-culture with primary retinal cells. Photoreceptor cell apoptosis accompanied mitochondrial apoptotic pathways, namely, activation of caspase-9 and translocation of apoptosis-inducing factor (AIF), from mitochondria to nuclei, as well as TUNEL-detectable DNA fragmentation. Finally, results from a mouse model of subretinal hemorrhage suggested that photoreceptor cells degenerated through the ligation of P2RX7 by extracellular ATP.

Though the number of experimental studies trying to decipher the changes triggered by SRH is limited, it is not questionable that severe tissue damage is induced both in an acute and chronic fashion. The studies have so far disclosed the damage that is related to the special situation of the subretinal space and the quite exquisite microarchitecture of the retina. However, more can be learned from studies analyzing the situation, changes, and tissue damage due to subarachnoid or intracerebral hematoma in the central nervous system (CNS) [14, 15]. Previous studies have found that several potential neurotoxic agents were released from extravascular blood, such as hemoglobin [16], iron [17] or glutamate [18], indicating that neurotoxic agents released from extravascular blood are the triggers of deleterious changes but can also be potential therapeutic targets. Besides the aspects of toxicity and initial mechanical forces that will irreversibly jeopardize visual acuity at an early stage, long-term function related to the central visual field will be significantly influenced by the size and exudative component of the resulting scar during the natural course.

Conclusion

In summary, SRH is a deleterious complication of different disease entities. The existing experimental studies show that tissue damage starts within the first hours but will significantly progress during the following days. Initially, mechanical factors such as hemorrhagic retinal detachment, shear forces, and clot contraction may be the major players responsible for the observed tissue damage. In the following both the barrier function of the clot, but more than this the toxic effect of some blood derived factors, such as iron, will initiate a degenerative cascade of the adjacent neurosensory tissue. Though irreversible damage will occur within the first days, the situation will continue to worsen due to the wound healing process associated with the hemorrhage. With respect to the natural course of SRH, a significant influence needs to be seen in the underlying disease. We need to understand that the observed changes in animal models are happening in an otherwise young and healthy environment. Preexisting damage, senescent tissue, as well as a progressing underlying disease, such as age-related macular degeneration, will for sure exert a considerably more prominent damage. As shown in the other chapters of this book related to etiopathology and clinical course, early action is advisable though functional results might be still limited. A special focus will be on the use of adjuvants to remove the SRH and its positive as well as potential toxic effect on the surrounding tissue. Though surgery is advisable, negative effects will result from mechanical forces and fluid dynamics applied during surgery for SRH removal.

References

1. Green WR, Key SM. Senile macular degeneration. A histopathological study. Trans Am Ophthalmol Soc. 1977;75:180–254.
2. Koshibu A. Ultrastructural studies on absorption of experimentally produced subretinal hemorrhage. I. Erythrophagocytosis at the early stage. Nippon Ganka Gakkai Zasshi. 1978;82:428–41.
3. Koshibu A. Ultrastructural studies on absorption of experimentally produced subretinal hemorrhage. II. Autolysis of macrophages and disappearance of erythrocytes from the subretinal space at the late stage. Nippon Ganka Gakkai Zasshi. 1978;82:471–9.
4. Koshibu A. Ultrastructural studies on absorption of experimentally produced subretinal hemorrhage. III. Absorption of erythrocyte breakdown products and retinal hemosiderosis at the late stage. Nippon Ganka Gakkai Zasshi. 1979;83:386–400.
5. Barber AN, Catsulis C, Cangelosi RJ. Studies on experimental retinitis. Light and electron microscopy. Br J Ophthalmol. 1971;55:91–105.
6. Burger PC, Klintworth GK. Experimental retinal degeneration in the rabbit produced by intraocular iron. Lab Invest. 1974;30:9–19.
7. Cibis PA, Yamashita T. Experimental aspects of ocular siderosis and hemosiderosis. Am J Ophthalmol. 1959;48:465–80.
8. Masciulli L, Anderson DR, Charles S. Experimental ocular siderosis in the squirrel monkey. Am J Ophthalmol. 1972;74:638–61.
9. Glatt H, Machemer R. Experimental subretinal hemorrhage in rabbits. Am J Ophthalmol. 1982;94:762–73.
10. Toth CA, Morse LS, Hjelmeland LM, Landers MB. Fibrin directs early retinal damage after experimental subretinal hemorrhage. Arch Ophthalmol. 1991;109:723–9.
11. Toth CA, Benner JD, Hjelmeland LM, Landers MB, Morse LS. Ultramicrosurgical removal of subretinal hemorrhage in cats. Am J Ophthalmol. 1992;113:175–82.
12. Bhisitkul RB, Winn BJ, Lee OT, Wong J, Pereira de S, Porco TC, He X, Hahn P, Dunaief JL. Neuroprotective effect of intravitreal triamcinolone acetonide against photoreceptor apoptosis in a rabbit model of subretinal hemorrhage. Invest Ophthalmol Vis Sci. 2008;49:4071–7.
13. Notomi S, Hisatomi T, Murakami Y, Terasaki H, Sonoda S, Asato R, Takeda A, Ikeda Y, Enaida H, Sakamoto T, Ishibashi T. Dynamic increase in extra-

cellular ATP accelerates photoreceptor cell apoptosis via ligation of P2RX7 in subretinal hemorrhage. PLoS One. 2013;8:e53338.
14. Hua Y, Keep RF, Hoff JT, Xi G. Brain injury after intracerebral hemorrhage: the role of thrombin and iron. Stroke. 2007;38:759–62.
15. Sacco RL, Wolf PA, Bharucha NE, Meeks SL, Kannel WB, et al. Subarachnoid and intracerebral hemorrhage: natural history, prognosis, and precursive factors in the Framingham Study. Neurology. 1984;34:847–54.
16. Regan RF, Panter SS. Hemoglobin potentiates excitotoxic injury in cortical cell culture. J Neurotrauma. 1996;13:223–31.
17. Nakamura T, Keep RF, Hua Y, Schallert T, Hoff JT, Xi G. Deferoxamine-induced attenuation of brain edema and neurological deficits in a rat model of intracerebral hemorrhage. J Neurosurg. 2004;100:672–8.
18. Qureshi AI, Ali Z, Suri MF, Shuaib A, Baker G, et al. Extracellular glutamate and other amino acids in experimental intracerebral hemorrhage: an in vivo microdialysis study. Crit Care Med. 2003;31:482–9.

2 Macular Haemorrhages: Natural Course and Risk Factors

Nicolas Feltgen

Introduction

Subretinal haemorrhage is a rare but serious complication that occurs in conjunction with macular diseases. The most common cause is choroidal neovascularisation (CNV) in the eyes with age-related macular degeneration (AMD). In some series, more than 80% of patients with submacular haemorrhage had underlying AMD [1, 2].

The different reasons for submacular haemorrhage can be divided into two subgroups [1, 3]: in the first, bleeding develops from a pre-existing CNV. This could be caused by AMD, myopia, presumed ocular histoplasmosis, angioid streaks, uveitis, laser treatment, or trauma or be idiopathic. CNV is absent in the second group. This condition can be found in association with retinal macroaneurysm, choroidal rupture, Valsalva manoeuvre, and Terson's syndrome.

The haemorrhage can be located under the retinal pigment epithelium (RPE), between the photoreceptors and the RPE, under the internal limiting membrane (ILM), or between ILM and vitreous. Blood in the retina's interior will usually resolve spontaneously and has a good prognosis, whereas the more common haemorrhage in the outer retinal segment has a poor prognosis.

N. Feltgen, MD
University Eye Hospital, Goettingen, Germany
e-mail: nicolas.feltgen@med.uni-goettingen.de

Pathophysiology

Subretinal haemorrhage is unfavourable for the retina, a factor attributable to four different pathways. First, the toxicity of iron in the blood causes irreversible damage to the retinal photoreceptors [4, 5]. Second, the mechanical barrier weakens the diffusion of nutrients between the retina and choroid (Fig. 2.1). Third, fibrin clotting leads to traction damage between the RPE and photoreceptors (Fig. 2.2), and fourth, the

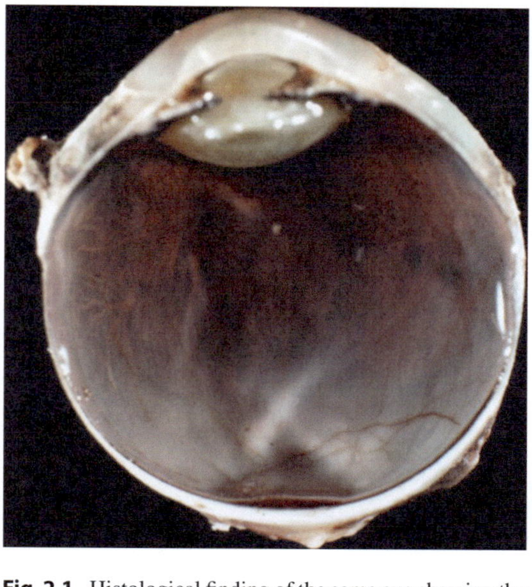

Fig. 2.1 Histological finding of the same eye showing the mechanical barrier, which compromises the photoreceptors' nutrition (HE staining, 12.5-fold magnification)

L.-O. Hattenbach (ed.), *Management of Macular Hemorrhage*,
https://doi.org/10.1007/978-3-319-65877-3_2

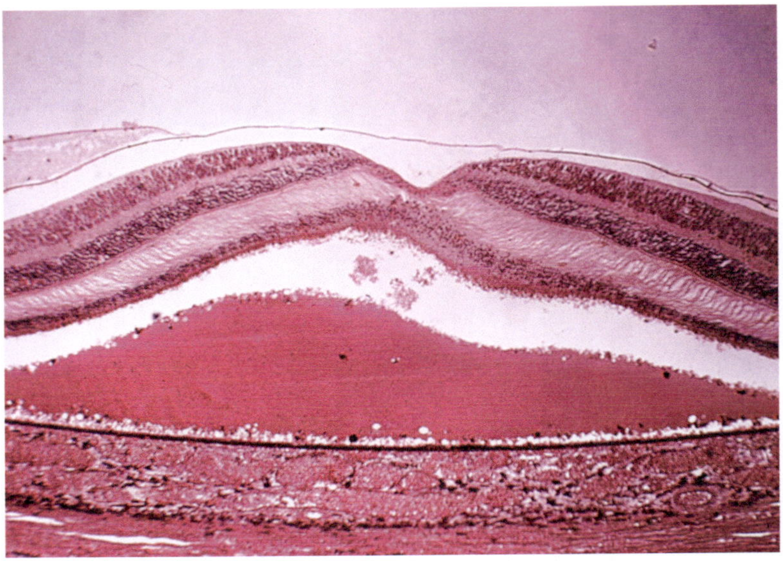

Fig. 2.2 Macroscopic finding of acute subretinal bleeding in a patient without AMD

triggered inflammation eventually leads to photoreceptor damage and the accumulation of macrophages [6–10]. The damage seems to correlate with the amount of bleeding [11].

Natural Course

The natural course of subretinal haemorrhage depends on the underlying disease, with CNV eyes having the poorest prognosis. Irreversible damage was detected within 24 h and a total loss of photoreceptors after 7 days in an animal model [4]. In eyes without CNV, the haemorrhage may resolve spontaneously without visible damage (Fig. 2.3).

In AMD patients, final best-corrected visual acuity (BCVA) ends between 20/2000 and 20/400, mean visual loss is 3.5 visual lines, and 75% of patients suffer significant visual loss of three lines or more (see Table 2.1).

The largest natural history study of submacular haemorrhage is the observation arm of the Submacular Surgery Trials Group B (B: Blood) who had predominantly haemorrhagic subfoveal neovascularisation associated with AMD [17]. That study included 168 patients ≥50 years with subretinal bleeding. Inclusion criteria were (1) subretinal haemorrhage with at least 50% of the CNV area being occupied by blood and (2) the entire lesion that did not exceed more than 3.5 disc areas. After 3 years, only 7 (8%) of the remaining 87 patients had a BCVA above 20/200, 16 (18%) eyes improved by at least two lines spontaneously, and BCVA decreased by two or more lines in 56 (64%) eyes. The median loss in BCVA over 3 years was 3.2 lines.

In conclusion, submacular haemorrhage is a condition that seriously threatens visual acuity, although spontaneous recovery has been observed in some patients. Patients experiencing spontaneous recovery usually have no underlying AMD, smaller haemorrhagic areas, and only a minimally elevated retina.

Recurrent Bleeding

The recurrence of macular bleeding was investigated by Hwang et al. in a retrospective analysis [18]. Of their 47 AMD patients presenting macular bleeding at their first visit, the incidence of recurrent submacular haemorrhage was 51% during the 3-year follow-up despite anti-VEGF treatment. The mean time for submacular haemorrhage to recur was 21.4 months. Polypoidal choroidal

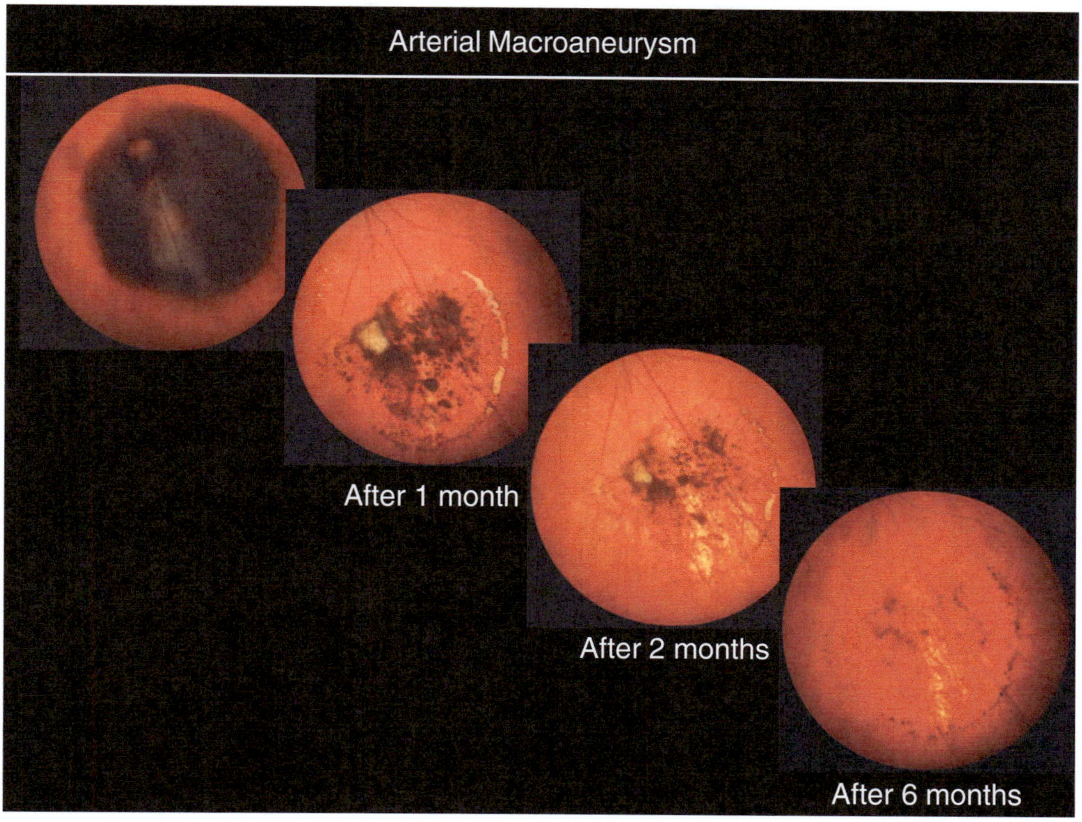

Fig. 2.3 Subretinal haemorrhage in an eye with arterial macroaneurysm in the periphery

Table 2.1 Clinical studies with submacular haemorrhage for different reasons

Author	Date	Design	Number of patients	Mean follow-up	Final BCVA	Comments
Bennett et al. [12]	1990	Retrospective	29	3 Years	20/480	• Prognosis poor with underlying AMD or bleeding thickness • Non-AMD eyes improved to 20/200
Berrocal et al. [13]	1996	Retrospective	31	2.5 Years	20/300	• Prognosis poor with underlying AMD
Avery et al. [14]	1996	Retrospective	40	3 Years	20/400	• Size and thickness correlated with visual outcome
Scupola et al. [15]	1999	Retrospective	54	2 Years	20/1250	• 90% of AMD eyes ≤20/200 • Size and thickness correlated with visual outcome
Chung et al. [16]	2001	Retrospective	12	4 Years	20/50	• Patients with BEST disease
SST group B report no. 13 [17]	2004	Prospective and randomised	168	3 Years	20/640	• Largest natural history study of AMD patients

vasculopathy was more often diagnosed in the group suffering from recurrent submacular bleeding.

Role of Systemic Disorders, Anticoagulant, and Antiplatelet Agents

There is little evidence in the literature on subretinal bleeding without choroidal or retinal diseases. Patients with systemic disorders like idiopathic thrombocytopenic purpura [19, 20], von Willebrand's disease [21], or haemophilia are described in some case reports [22]. An increasing problem correlating with submacular haemorrhage in AMD patients might be their concurrent use of anticoagulant or antiplatelet agents. In the prospective SST Group B trial, 26% of all patients had taken warfarin and 32% took aspirin daily [17]. Some case reports have suggested a negative impact from anticoagulants on the clinical course of AMD patients [23–28]. This impression was confirmed in clinical studies: in the retrospective study of Kuhli-Hattenbach et al., patients taking anticoagulants or antiplatelet agents exhibited a more extensive subretinal haemorrhage area than patients not taking blood thinners [29]. Others have reported this correlation also: the relative risk of bleeding is increased fourfold [30–32]. With the concurrent use of warfarin, the annual incidence of subretinal haemorrhage rises from 0.04 to 0.1% [30, 32, 33]. On the other hand, patients taking anticoagulants or antiplatelet agents usually have serious systemic vascular diseases needing treatment. It is not surprising that patients with high blood pressure reveal more extensive subretinal bleeding.

References

1. Bopp S. [Subretinal hemorrhage. Natural course and staging]. Ophthalmologica. 2012;109:635–43.
2. Ibanez HE, Williams DF, Thomas MA, Ruby AJ, Meredith TA, Boniuk I, Grand MG. Surgical management of submacular hemorrhage. A series of 47 consecutive cases. Arch Ophthalmol. 1995;113:62–9.
3. Hochman MA, Seery CM, Zarbin MA. Pathophysiology and management of subretinal hemorrhage. Surv Ophthalmol. 1997;42:195–213.
4. Glatt H, Machemer R. Experimental subretinal hemorrhage in rabbits. Am J Ophthalmol. 1982;94:762–73.
5. Koshibu A. [Ultrastructural studies on absorption of an experimentally produced subretinal hemorrhage. III. Absorption of erythrocyte break down products and retinal hemosiderosis at the late stage (author's transl)]. Nippon Ganka Gakkai Zasshi. 1979;83:386–400.
6. Dastgheib K, Green WR. Granulomatous reaction to Bruch's membrane in age-related macular degeneration. Arch Ophthalmol. 1994;1960(112):813–8.
7. El Baba F, Jarrett WH, Harbin TS, Fine SL, Michels RG, Schachat AP, Green WR. Massive hemorrhage complicating age-related macular degeneration. Clinicopathologic correlation and role of anticoagulants. Ophthalmology. 1986;93:1581–92.
8. Reynders S, Lafaut BA, Aisenbrey S, Broecke CV, Lucke K, Walter P, Kirchhof B, Bartz-Schmidt KU. Clinicopathologic correlation in hemorrhagic age-related macular degeneration. Graefes Arch Clin Exp Ophthalmol. 2002;240:279–85.
9. Toth CA, Morse LS, Hjelmeland LM, Landers MB. Fibrin directs early retinal damage after experimental subretinal hemorrhage. Arch Ophthalmol. 1991;1960(109):723–9.
10. Wolter JR, Till GO. Multinucleated giant cells on Bruch's membrane late in recurrent retinal and subretinal hemorrhaging. Ophthalmologica. 1989;199:53–9.
11. Stanescu-Segall D, Balta F, Jackson TL. Submacular hemorrhage in neovascular age-related macular degeneration: a synthesis of the literature. Surv Ophthalmol. 2016;61:18–32.
12. Bennett SR, Folk JC, Blodi CF, Klugman M. Factors prognostic of visual outcome in patients with subretinal hemorrhage. Am J Ophthalmol. 1990;109:33–7.
13. Berrocal MH, Lewis ML, Flynn HW. Variations in the clinical course of submacular hemorrhage. Am J Ophthalmol. 1996;122:486–93.
14. Avery RL, Fekrat S, Hawkins BS, Bressler NM. Natural history of subfoveal subretinal hemorrhage in age-related macular degeneration. Retina. 1996;16:183–9.
15. Scupola A, Coscas G, Soubrane G, Balestrazzi E. Natural history of macular subretinal hemorrhage in age-related macular degeneration. Ophthalmologica. 1999;213:97–102.
16. Chung MM, Oh KT, Streb LM, Kimura AE, Stone EM. Visual outcome following subretinal hemorrhage in Best disease. Retina. 2001;21:575–80.
17. Bressler NM, Bressler SB, Childs AL, Haller JA, Hawkins BS, Lewis H, MacCumber MW, Marsh MJ, Redford M, Sternberg P, Thomas MA, Williams GA, Submacular Surgery Trials (SST) Research Group. Surgery for hemorrhagic choroidal neovascular lesions of age-related macular degeneration: ophthalmic findings: SST report no. 13. Ophthalmology. 2004;111:1993–2006.

18. Hwang J-U, Yang SJ, Yoon YH, Lee JY, Kim J-G. Recurrent submacular hemorrhage in patients with neovascular age-related macular degeneration. Retina. 2012;32:652–7.
19. Okuda A, Inoue M, Shinoda K, Tsubota K. Massive bilateral vitreoretinal hemorrhage in patient with chronic refractory idiopathic thrombocytopenic purpura. Graefes Arch Clin Exp Ophthalmol. 2005; 243:1190–3.
20. Shah PA, Yang SS, Fung WE. Idiopathic thrombocytopenic purpura with massive subretinal hemorrhage. Arch Ophthalmol. 2005;1960(123):1612–3.
21. Herrmann WA, Lohmann CP, Demmler-Hackenberg M, Gabel V-P. Von Willebrand's disease type I as a cause for subvitreal, retinal and subretinal haemorrhages. Graefes Arch Clin Exp Ophthalmol. 2005;243:383–5.
22. Wang T-Y, Horng C-T, Cheng S-N, Li C-H, Chen J-T, Tsai M-L. Optic disc hemorrhages in a patient with hemophilia A. Int J Hematol. 2008;87:550–2.
23. Brown GC, Tasman WS, Shields JA. Massive subretinal hemorrhage and anticoagulant therapy. Can J Ophthalmol. 1982;17:227–30.
24. Caronia RM, Sturm RT, Fastenberg DM, Berke SJ, Weintraub J. Bilateral secondary angle-closure glaucoma as a complication of anticoagulation in a nanophthalmic patient. Am J Ophthalmol. 1998;126:307–9.
25. Daus W, Völcker HE. [Clinical aspects, differential diagnosis and histopathology of spontaneous subretinal mass hemorrhage]. Klin Monbl Augenheilkd. 1991;199:16–21.
26. Knox FA, Johnston PB. Spontaneous suprachoroidal haemorrhage in a patient with age-related macular degeneration on excessive anticoagulation therapy. Eye (Lond). 2002;16:669–70.
27. Lewis H, Sloan SH, Foos RY. Massive intraocular hemorrhage associated with anticoagulation and age-related macular degeneration. Graefes Arch Clin Exp Ophthalmol. 1988;226:59–64.
28. Weir CR, Nolan DJ, Holding D, Hammer H. Intraocular haemorrhage associated with anticoagulant therapy. Acta Ophthalmol Scand. 2000; 78:492–3.
29. Kuhli-Hattenbach C, Fischer IB, Schalnus R, Hattenbach L-O. Subretinal hemorrhages associated with age-related macular degeneration in patients receiving anticoagulation or antiplatelet therapy. Am J Ophthalmol. 2010;149:316–321.e1.
30. Kiernan DF, Hariprasad SM, Rusu IM, Mehta SV, Mieler WF, Jager RD. Epidemiology of the association between anticoagulants and intraocular hemorrhage in patients with neovascular age-related macular degeneration. Retina. 2010;30:1573–8.
31. Kingham JD, Chen MC, Levy MH. Macular hemorrhage in the aging eye: the effects of anticoagulants. N Engl J Med. 1988;318:1126–7.
32. Tilanus MA, Vaandrager W, Cuypers MH, Verbeek AM, Hoyng CB. Relationship between anticoagulant medication and massive intraocular hemorrhage in age-related macular degeneration. Graefes Arch Clin Exp Ophthalmol. 2000;238:482–5.
33. Kuhli-Hattenbach C, Miesbach W, Scharrer I, Hattenbach L-O. [Massive subretinal hemorrhage and anticoagulants. An unfortunate combination?]. Ophthalmologica. 2012;109:665–9.

Classification of Macular Hemorrhages

3

Silvia Bopp and Alireza Mirshahi

Introduction

Macular hemorrhages are a complication of various diseases [1, 2]. They arise either from the choroidal or the retinal circulation. Most commonly, the underlying pathology is a choroidal neovascular membrane (CNVM), especially in AMD patients. Less common ocular diseases are those with non-AMD-related CNVM and retinal arterial macroaneurysms (RAM) [3]. Dependent on the location (sub-, intra-, preretinal), the prognosis varies considerably. In particular, the natural history studies demonstrate a poor prognosis for subfoveal hemorrhages; however, a significant portion of the eyes may have a favorable outcome [4]. Therefore, therapeutic decision-making is difficult in the individual case.

A major difficulty in comparing different treatment modalities for macular hemorrhages is the lack of a standardized definition of the extent and location of the blood. Earlier studies on this issue graded subretinal macular hemorrhages according to the size (small, large) and the thickness (flat, moderate, thick), but fundus and FAG/ICG tools did not allow a further differentiation [5, 6]. We are now aware that additional criteria affect the prognosis and therapeutic approach. Current imaging techniques allow a much more precise description of the individual pathology. New classifications for non-hemorrhagic AMD have been suggested and take into account the improved diagnostic tools [7]

Even more complex is the situation in the eyes with macular hemorrhages. In face of the fact that the prognosis is variable, a lot of treatment strategies have been suggested. There is an ongoing controversy when to treat and how to treat. As patient cohorts and treatment modalities are highly heterogeneous, no reliable comparative data is available on outcomes. Thus, as a first step for such studies, the authors suggest a classification for macular hemorrhages including their size, thickness, and intraretinal location taking into account the clinical presentation and current imaging techniques. Most parameters can be adopted for macular hemorrhages of other causes than CNVM- and RAM-related macular bleedings.

Clinical Presentation of Macular Hemorrhages

Macular hemorrhages can cause devastating visual loss [6]. Most often, elderly patients with age-related macular degeneration are affected, followed by patients with retinal arterial

S. Bopp, MD (✉)
Eye Clinic Universitätsallee, Bremen, Germany
e-mail: s.bopp@retina.to

A. Mirshahi, MD
Dardenne Eye Hospital, Bonn, Germany

L.-O. Hattenbach (ed.), *Management of Macular Hemorrhage*,
https://doi.org/10.1007/978-3-319-65877-3_3

macroaneurysms. Other conditions that can cause macular hemorrhages are PCV (polypoidal choroidal vasculopathy), secondary CNVMs of various origin, posttraumatic choroidal ruptures, Valsalva-maculopathy, and Terson's syndrome. Basically, the source of bleeding that affects the macula is the choroidal or retinal vasculature. Thus, hemorrhages may be located sub-, intra-, and preretinally (sub-ILM, subhyaloidal). Determination of the location of blood is essential, as this is the major factor with regard to visual prognosis. Today's imaging techniques are helpful and allow a distinct differentiation. Furthermore, preexisting or associated pathologies affect the prognosis, for instance, a subfoveal CNVM or a choroidal rupture. Thus, the knowledge of the natural course of the underlying disease and the location and amount of blood are the major criteria on which therapeutic decisions are based on. It is commonly agreed that in particular subretinal hemorrhages have the most dubious prognosis and the motivation to seek for appropriate therapies, because the natural history is expected to be poor [6] (Figs. 3.1, 3.2, and 3.3).

Premacular Hemorrhages

Bleeding that originates from the retinal vasculature or retinal neovascularizations usually speeds under the ILM or in the subhyaloidal space or even into the vitreous cavity. Most commonly these types of hemorrhage occur in diabetic retinopathy and other vasoproliferative diseases, in which new vessels are the source of bleeding. More rarely Valsalva maneuvers and Terson's syndrome may lead to macular hemorrhages. Pathogenetically a high intravasal pressure of retinal or peripapillary vessels is causative for the bleeding. As the subretinal space is not affected, prognosis for preretinal hemorrhages is favourable, both with and without treatment (Figs. 3.1 and 3.2).

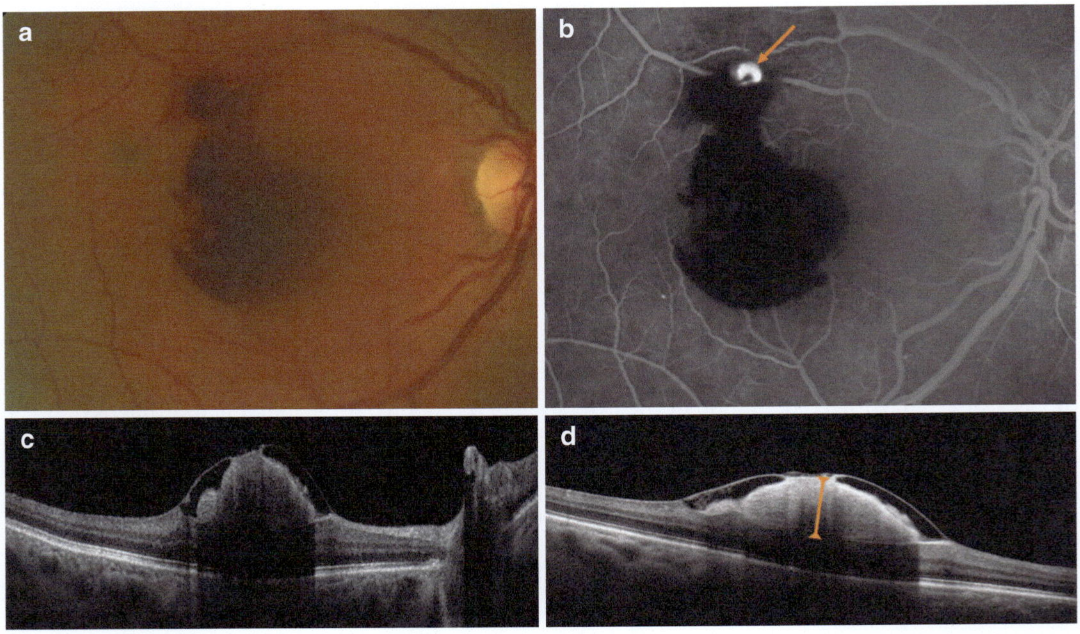

Fig. 3.1 Preretinal macular hemorrhage due to a ruptured retinal arterial macroaneurysm (RAM): (**a**) Fundus photography reveals a preretinal hemorrhage with adjacent vitreous involvement. (**b**) By FAG, the retinal vessels are obscured by blood, but a distinct hyperfluorescent arterial ectasia is outlined characteristic for an active RAM. (**c**) SD-OCT shows a hyperreflective mass and a separation of the ILM. (**d**) Enhanced HD OCT also shows a homogenous clot and that the retinal layers appear to be normal, thickness of the hemorrhage 400 μm (bar). FLATCAPS classification: F1 L0 A0 T0 P0 S1. *Clinical significance*: Immediate surgical removal is not indicated, as there is obviously no subretinal blood component

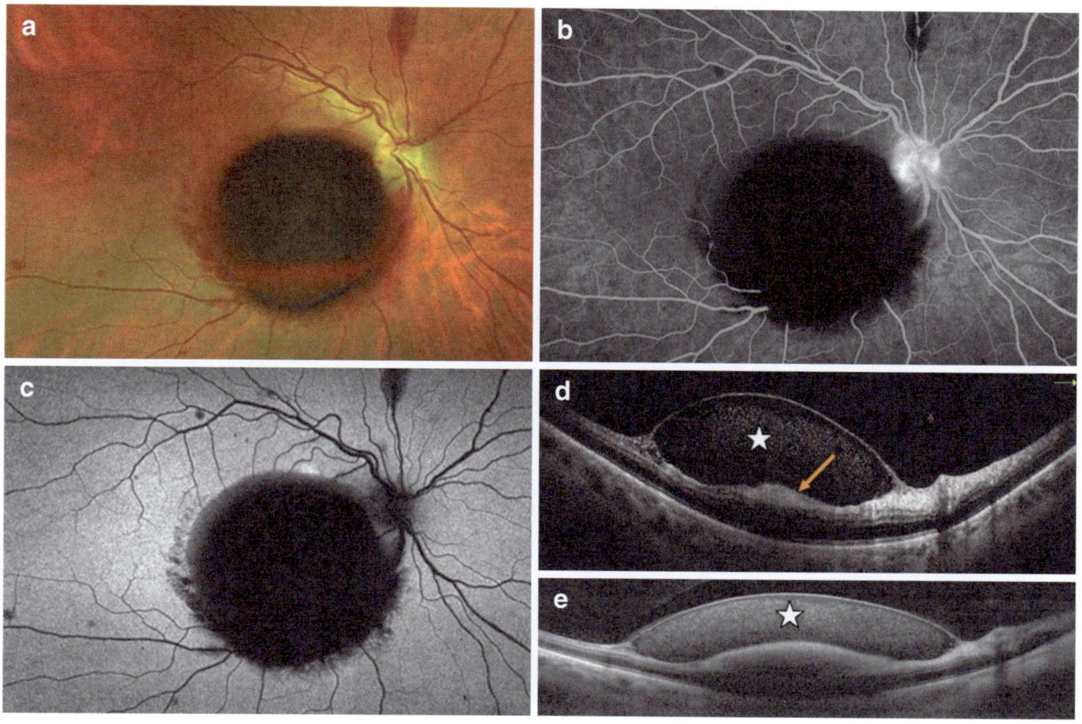

Fig. 3.2 Preretinal macular hemorrhage (hypertensive crisis): (**a**) Fundus image reveals a preretinal hemorrhage with an inferior sedimentation of blood. (**b**) FAG shows complete blockage of retinal vessels. (**c**) FAF reveals no RPE anomalies. (**d, e**) Wide-angle OCT imaging depicts a cystic elevation of the ILM filled with lysed blood (asterisk), possibly clotted close to the retina (arrow), the retinal layers so not seem to be affected. FLATCAPS classification: F1 L0 A1 T1 P0 S2. *Clinical significance*: Immediate surgical removal is not indicated, as there is obviously no subretinal blood component. To enhance blood resorption, laser hyaloidotomy can be considered as the ILM is distant from the macula

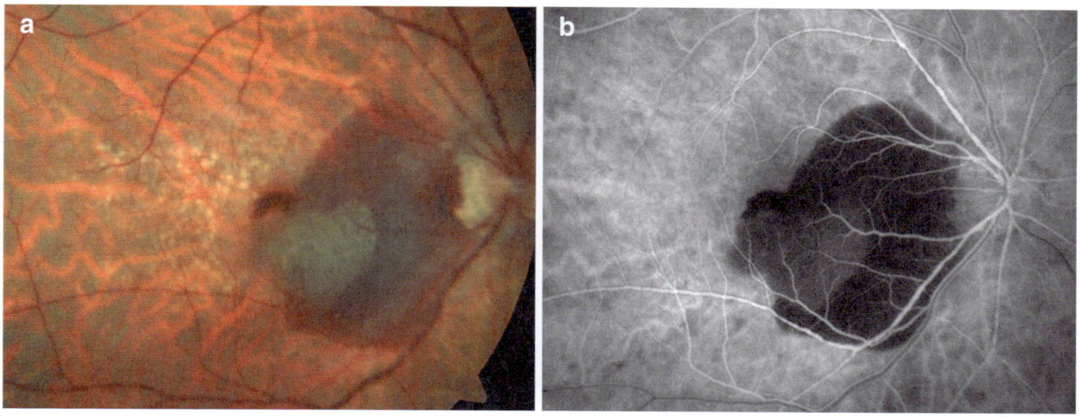

Fig. 3.3 Macular hemorrhage in AMD: (**a**) Color fundus photography reveals a subretinal hemorrhage in the papillomacular area with a grayish and reddish aspect. (**b**) By FAG, subretinal and choroidal structures are obscured, and no leakage is observed in the late phase. (**c**) FAF shows a normal RPE pattern centrally (asterisk), but adjacent subretinal blood obscures the background fluorescence (arrow). (**d, e**) In SD-OCT the fovea is only just involved by the hemorrhage. Sub-RPE and subretinal blood can be distinguished (bars). Subfoveal blood thickness is about 250 µm. FLATCAPS classification: F1 L3 A1 T0 P1 S1. *Clinical significance*: anti-VEGF monotherapy only may be successful

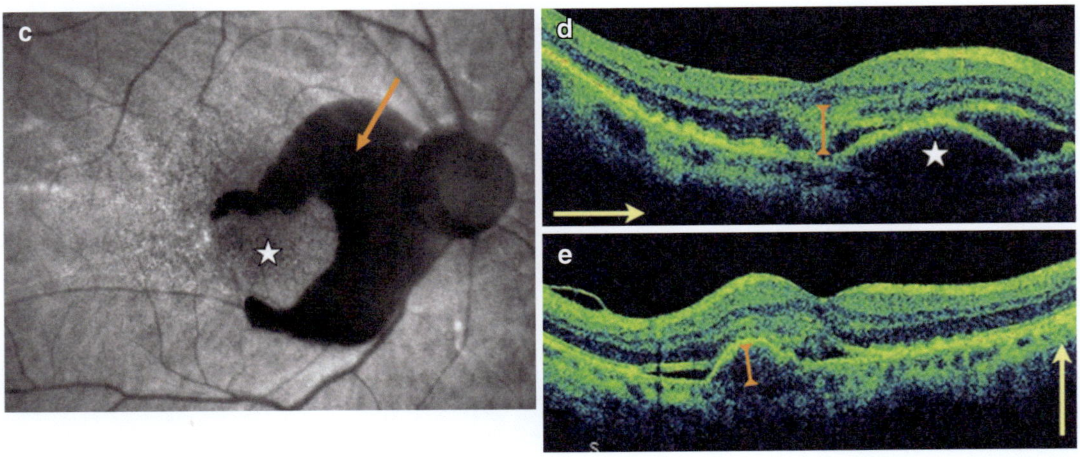

Fig. 3.3 (continued)

Subretinal Hemorrhages

Basically, subretinal hemorrhages occur with or without a CNVM. The vast majority are CNVM-related AMD cases (approximately 90%). From those type 2 (occult type, pigment epithelial detachment), type 3 (retinal angiomatous proliferation, RAP), and type 4 (PCV) carry the greatest risk to develop hemorrhagic complications. Rarely, this happens in non-AMD-related CNVM, such as myopic and posttraumatic cases. The source of bleeding is the pathologic vasculature of the CNVM that originates from the choroid (Figs. 3.3–3.6).

In up to 10%, a retinal arterial macroaneurysm is the cause of subretinal hemorrhage and not associated with a CNVM. Differential diagnosis to hemorrhagic AMD may be difficult, if the blood is predominantly in the subretinal space. However, many cases present with a mixed-type of bleeding, therefore showing also pre- and intraretinal blood components. In contrast to AMD-related hemorrhages, the source of bleeding is a rupture of a retinal artery. As a result of the high intravasal pressure, the extension of blood does not respect the natural horizontal barriers of the retina but spreads anteriorly toward the vitreoretinal interface and vitreous body and/or to the subretinal space. In very few cases the cause of a subretinal hemorrhage is initially uncertain and becomes evident later in the course (Fig. 3.5).

Why Is There a Need for a Classification?

The cause of the bleeding is one of the most important prognostic factors of macular hemorrhages [1, 4]. While bleedings related to age-related macular degeneration (AMD) have a guarded prognosis, macular hemorrhages secondary to retinal macroaneurysms or a choroidal rupture have a better visual outcome. Other decisive factors are the extent of the hemorrhage, its thickness, and its location in relation to the fovea. The damage to the central vision is caused by the complex pathological processes at the level of choriocapillaris, retinal pigment epithelium, and photoreceptors or by the blood itself [8, 9] (also see Chapters (1) Pathophysiology of Macular Hemorrhages and (2) Natural Course and Risk Factors). A classification of macular hemorrhages should help clinicians in several ways: (1) by considering the abovementioned prognostic factors, the classification will enable the clinician to assess the potential outcome of the bleeding and give a realistic expectation to the patients, and (2) the classification will help the retinal surgeon in choosing the most appropriate treatment strategy in each case, e.g., a rather small, thin

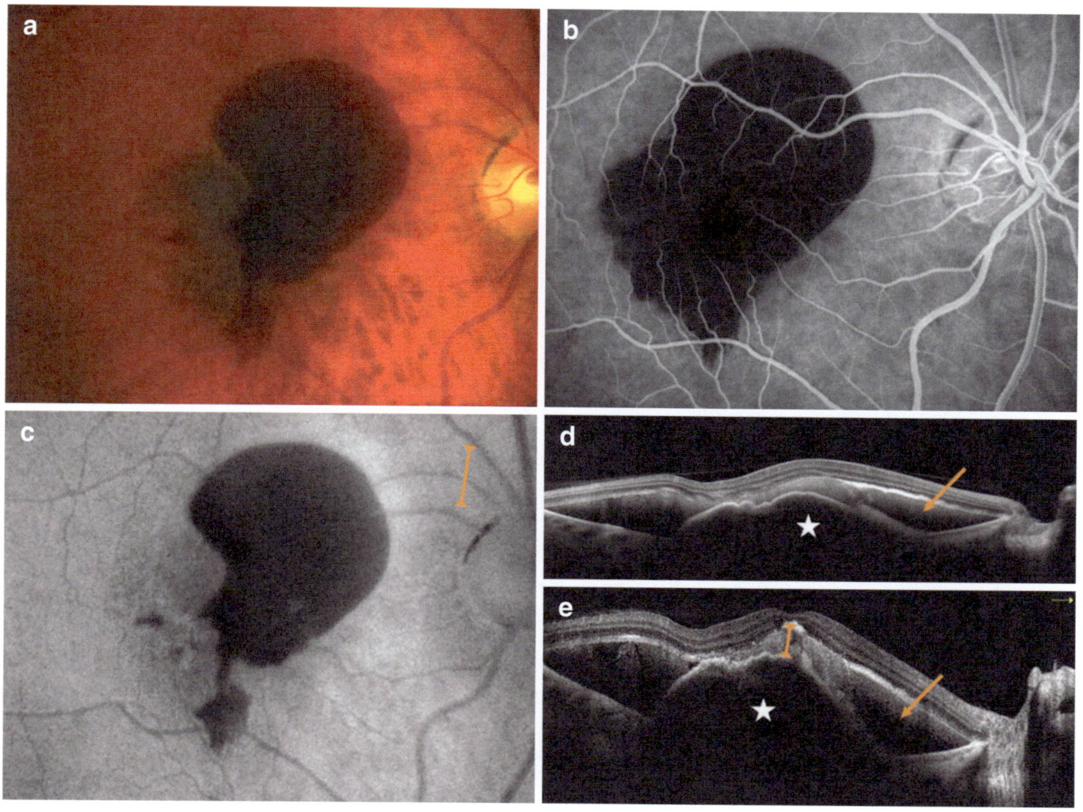

Fig. 3.4 AMD-related subretinal hemorrhage: (**a**) Fundus photography reveals a subretinal hemorrhage temporally darker than nasally. (**b**) By FAG, retinal vessels appear normal, but choroidal structures are obscured by blood, and no hyperfluorescence typical for an occult CNVM can be seen. (**c**) FAF shows a normal RPE pattern in the temporal part of the hemorrhage indicative for a sub-RPE blood component. (**d**) In enhanced HD-OCT imaging, blood can be detected in the subretinal space (arrows), and a large PED is present (asterisks). (**e**) SD-OCT shows similar findings and the macula attached to the hyperreflective blood clot, subfoveal blood thickness is 300 μm (bar). FLATCAPS classification: F1 L3 A0 T0 P1 S1. *Clinical significance*: Example for a case in which medical or surgical treatment is discussed controversially. The subretinal component is flat only, but a significant hemorrhagic PED is present

submacular hemorrhage secondary to AMD, and sparing the fovea might be best treated by intravitreal anti-VEGF drugs [10] while the same hemorrhage involving the fovea, a rather aggressive treatment option may be appropriate, such as subretinal r-TPA and anti-VEGF injection and gas tamponade [11] (see following chapters).

Last but not least, a classification will help clinicians in comparing their outcome results of different treatment strategies. Since the visual outcome is related both to the initial situation and the chosen therapy, a classification will facilitates in assessing the efficacy and safety of any treatment in a certain type of macular hemorrhage.

FLATCAPS Classification System for Macular Hemorrhages: (Foveal Involvement, Layer, Age, Thickness, Cause/Pathogenesis, Size)

In the following, we present the FLATCAPS classification for macular hemorrhages. It includes the following criteria: size of the hemorrhage, the pathogenetic cause, the thickness, its age and duration, as well as foveal involvement. Multimodal imaging is mandatory to describe the individual pathoanatomic situation. Table 3.1 summarizes the FLATCAPS classification system.

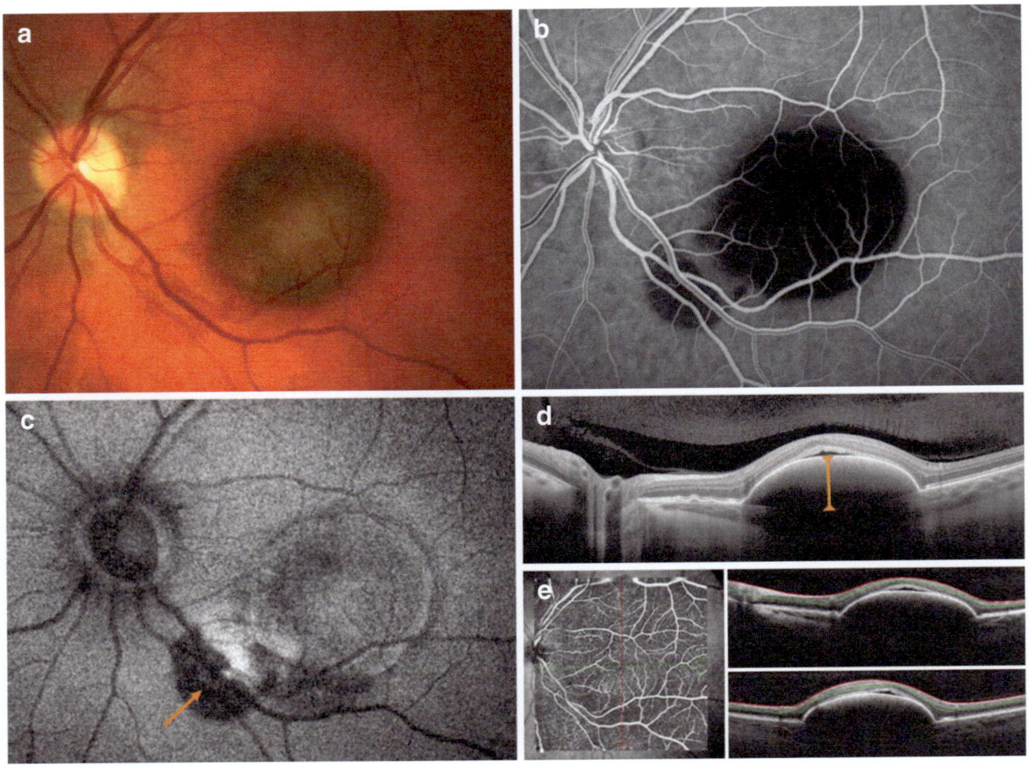

Fig. 3.5 Sub-RPE hemorrhage of uncertain cause (45-year-old female): (**a**) Fundus photography reveals a red-grayish subretinal hemorrhage. (**b**) By FAG, the retinal vessels are normal; subretinal and choroidal structures are completely obscured. (**c**) FAF shows the margins of the hemorrhagic lesion, but RPE is not much altered. Inferonasally a subretinal blood component is present (arrow). (**d**) In enhanced HD-OCT, a bullous RPE detachment with minor internal reflectivity is present and a small subfoveal dehiscence; thickness of the hemorrhage is estimated about 600 μm (bar). (**e**) OCT-A shows a normal retinal flow, but segmentation does not allow to judge a possible sub-RPE vascular pathology. FLATCAPS classification: F1 L2 A2 T1 P0 or P1 (uncertain) S1. *Clinical significance*: ICG angiography may help to establish the diagnosis (vascular PED? PCV?). Symptomatic blood displacement would not work in this case and carries a high risk to result in a RPE rip

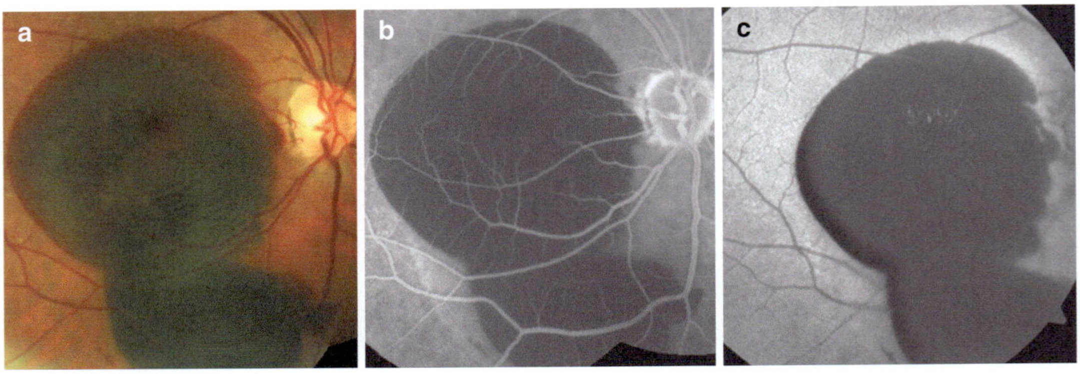

Fig. 3.6 AMD-related subretinal mass hemorrhage: (**a**) Fundus photography reveals a prominent homogeneously appearing subretinal hemorrhage exceeding the inferior vessel arcade. (**b**) By FAG, choroidal structures are obscured by blood, and no hyperfluorescent spot typical for a CNVM can be detected. (**c**) In FAF, no RPE structures could be detected within the lesion due to a complete blockage. (**d**) En face OCT and OCT map give information of the deeper structures (homogeneous blood clot) and a normal retinal thickness overlying the bulky hemorrhage. (**e**) SD-OCT shows a prominent subretinal mass bleeding (asterisk) of >1000 μm (bar). The shadowing effect does not allow a precise judgment about the extent of a possible RPE detachment (arrow). FLATCAPS classification: F1 L1 A0 T2 P1 S3. *Clinical significance*: most likely, an indication for subretinal surgery

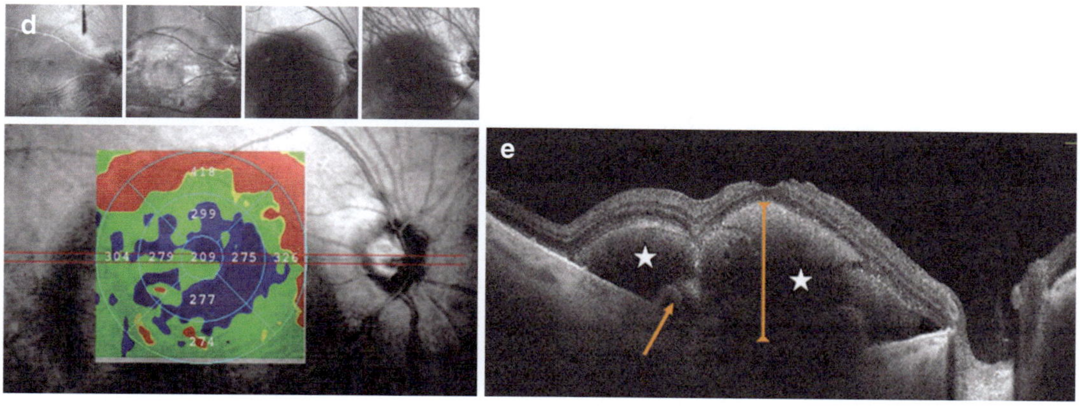

Fig. 3.6 (continued)

Table 3.1 FLATCAPS classification system for macular hemorrhages (foveal involvement, layer, age, thickness, cause/pathogenesis, size)

		Comments for the clinician
1. Foveal involvement		
F0	No	Observation or treatment of the causative disease
F1	Yes	Consider treatment of the macular hemorrhage
2. Retinal layers		
L0	Preretinal (subhyaloidal/ sub-ILM)	Vitrectomy if no absorption and foveal involvement, laser hyaloidotomy in certain cases
L1	Subretinal	Consider blood displacement strategies for subfoveal thick bleedings
L2	sub-RPE	Attention: blood dislocation may be ineffective, RPE-rip
L3	Mixed subretinal and sub-RPE	The subretinal part can be displaced by surgery, but not the sub-RPE component
L4	Blood present in more than two retinal layers mentioned above	Typical for retinal macroaneurysms
3. Age/duration[a]		
A0	Up to 7 days	L1–4: based on experimental finding, best prognosis after surgery
A1	8–14 days	L1–4: no solid data whether the prognosis is worse compared to A0
A2	Older than 2 weeks	Guarded prognosis, iron toxicity
4. Thickness		
T0	<500 μm	L1–4: anti-VEGF and subretinal surgery work well, superiority of either method is not investigated
T1	500–1000 μm	L1–4: is generally considered an indication for surgery
T2	>1000 μm	Poor prognosis, consider “maximal” surgery
5. Cause/pathogenesis		
P0	Non-neovascular	Good visual prognosis
P1	Neovascular (choroidal)	Additional and continuous treatment of the CNVM (e.g., anti-VEGF) mandatory
P2	Neovascular (retinal)	Grading and treatment of the underlying disease
6. Size[a]		
S0	<1 DA	L1–4: rarely requires surgical intervention
S1	1–5 DA	L1–4: surgery is considered to be useful in F1
S2	>5 DA and up to the arcades	L1–4: indication for surgery, but best technique not known
S3	Massive hemorrhage exceeding the arcades	Individual decision-making, possibly extensive surgery to preserve some vision

AMD age-related macular degeneration, *CNVM* choroidal neovascular membrane, *DA* disc area, *ILM* internal limiting membrane, *PCV* polypoidal choroidal vasculopathy, *RAP* retinal angiomatous proliferation, *RPE* retinal pigment epithelium

[a]Is of prognostic significance, if the blood is located subretinally, but less critical in conditions with preretinal hemorrhages

Foveal Involvement

F0 Non
F1 Yes

Rationale: The visual acuity is not jeopardized when the bleeding does not involve the fovea. The hemorrhage will resolve by time when its cause is non-neovascular. Even if the cause is a choroidal neovascular membrane, anti-VEGF intravitreal injections alone have shown a favorable outcome in small hemorrhagic lesions [10]. One should weigh the risks of any surgical treatment carefully when the bleeding does not include the central retina against its benefits. The authors have observed cases, performed elsewhere, in which the para-macular blood has been displaced to subfoveal area by intravitreal recombinant tissue plasminogen activator (TPA) and gas resulting in severe deterioration of visual acuity. Therefore, one should be cautious in aggressively treating non-foveal subretinal hemorrhages. Reversely, the authors believe that the expected blood/iron toxicity to the central retina justifies a proactive surgical treatment of subretinal hemorrhages should the fovea be involved. Nonetheless, other classification criteria must be considered in the decision-making process.

Layers Involved

L0: preretinal (subhyaloidal/sub-ILM)
L1: subretinal
L2: sub-RPE
L3: mixed subretinal and sub-RPE
L4: blood present in more than two spaces mentioned above

Rationale: Identifying the layer(s) involved in the hemorrhage is crucial for the choice of treatment. Clinical investigation, fluorescein angiography, and optical coherence tomography (OCT) help clinicians in identifying the exact location of the bleeding [9]. Preretinal hemorrhages including the subhyaloidal and sub-internal limiting membrane (ILM) space can be treated by pars plana vitrectomy (PPV) [12]. In case of a sub-ILM bleeding, removal of the blood may require surgical peeling of the ILM to get access to the blood. In case of a prominent subhyaloidal hemorrhage, laser treatment (hyaloidotomy either with Nd:YAG or argon laser) may be helpful in relieving the blood into the vitreous cavity where resorption occurs more rapidly and allows identification of the cause and a possible submacular involvement (F0, F1 classification).

Exclusive subretinal bleedings (L1) are best candidates for any strategy targeting blood displacement (including intravitreal or subretinal r-TPA and gas injection). However, surgical treatment of predominantly sub-RPE hemorrhages (L2) that can be observed in AMD cases is less successful in our experience either as there is limited access of the drug to the sub-RPE layer or, more likely, for anatomic reasons, as there is no preformed horizontal structure like the subretinal space (between photoreceptorouter segments and RPE) where the blood could be displaced easily. As those cases often present with an additional subretinal component (L3 classification), we observe after surgical interventions aiming at blood displacement that the subretinal component may move away sufficiently, but the sub-RPE component remains. L3 classification refers to a condition when blood can be identified partially in the subretinal and in parts under the RPE. Cautious assessment of the OCT, fundus imaging using color and blue filter, and fluorescein angiography are mandatory to detect and distinguish sub-RPE from subretinal bleeding. In fundus photographs blood under the RPE appears darker than subretinal hemorrhage. Bleedings secondary to a retinal macroaneurysm may be present in more than two layers mentioned above; thus, whenever blood is detected in several retinal layers with the center of the hemorrhage close to a retinal artery, a macroaneurysm should be considered as a probable cause (L4 classification).

Age/Duration

A0: up to 7 days
A1: 8–14 days
A2: older than 2 weeks

Rationale: Many surgeons intend to operate on submacular hemorrhages within a week of their occurrence. The rationale of early intervention is based on the fact that irreversible iron toxicity to the retina is to be expected early when photoreceptor cells are in direct conjunction with the blood [8, 13]. Hemorrhages older than 2 weeks are thought to have a more limited visual outcome due to the aforementioned reasons and further pathological tissue reaction, such as inflammation and insufficient nutrition to the outer retina (A2 classification). We do not know whether there is a difference in visual outcome between the A0 and A1 groups; however, the classification should encourage and enable clinical researchers to find an answer in future studies.

Thickness

T1: <500 μm
T2: 500–1000 μm
T3: >1000 μm

Rationale: The hemorrhage thickness is related to its visual outcome prognosis: Thin subretinal bleedings have a good and realistic chance to be resolved within a few weeks spontaneously or with intravitreal medication and may also do well after been displaced by intravitreal or subretinal r-TPA injection and gas. Very thick hemorrhages [9, 14] tend to last for several months in their natural course and are less responsive to surgical displacement strategies. Furthermore, intravitreal anti-VEGF drugs may not sufficiently get access to the choroidal neovascular membrane (CNVM) in cases of large and particularly thick (T3 type) hemorrhages. The authors believe that considering very large (S3) and thick (T3) bleedings involving the fovea (F1) particularly originating from a choroidal neovascularization (P1) may be candidates for "maximal" surgery, including 360° retinotomy with or without macular translocation [15, 16]. Thickness measurements are performed with OCT imaging: point of reference can be the foveal center or the maximal clot thickness elsewhere.

Cause/Pathogenesis

P0: Non-neovascular
P1: Neovascular (choroidal)
P2: Neovascular (retinal)

Rationale: The underlying disease and initial pathoanatomic situation that has led to a macular hemorrhage are of crucial importance for the visual prognosis and treatment strategy [1, 4, 17]. Bleedings secondary to non-neovascular conditions, e.g., retinal macroaneurysm, have a better outcome when the blood has been displaced surgically than those secondary to a CNVM.

Clinicians must consider the cause of bleeding to decide upon the initial and possible further treatment strategy. If a choroidal neovascular membrane is the cause, anti-VEGF-medication should be added to any treatment regimen, either at the time of primary intervention or shortly thereafter. Since submacular hemorrhages secondary to age-related macular degeneration (AMD) or polypoidal choroidal vasculopathy (PCV) tend to recur a proactive and continuous anti-VEGF regime may be mandatory. Repeated intravitreal injections with anti-VEGF drugs will help in maintaining the visual improvement gained with the initial blood displacing surgical therapy. Retinal neovascularization in proliferative diabetic retinopathy may result in pre- and intraretinal hemorrhages that may affect the posterior pole and is possibly the leading symptom for the patient. However, it occurs among various other fundus findings. Treatment here depends on the severity of retinopathy as a whole (NPDR, PDR, with/without macular edema, pucker, etc.)

Size

S0: <1 Disc area (DA)
S1: 1–5 DA
S2: >5 DA and up to the arcades
S3: Massive hemorrhage exceeding the arcades

Rationale: The extent of hemorrhage, in particular when located subretinally, is an important prognostic factor. Small hemorrhages [18, 19] rarely require surgical intervention (S0 type). The natural course of large and massive hemorrhages (S2 and S3) is dubious, particularly if thick clots (T3 type) are present. Therefore, the visual outcome which is to be expected in the natural course and the risk/benefit ratio with invasive surgical maneuvers should be discussed with the individual patient, especially when rather invasive surgical treatments (including peripheral retinotomies, subretinal blood lavage with/without 360° macular translocation) are offered [15]. Moderate-sized hemorrhages (S1) need intervention, particularly if they involve the fovea (F1). Which kind of treatment—either intravitreal medication or vitreoretinal surgery—is largely controversial. Up to now, there is no solid data whether these eyes do better with anti-VEGF or with the one or other surgical technique. Other classification criteria should be considered in addition to the size when assessing the necessity and kind of surgical treatment.

Conclusion

The proposed FLATCAPS classification of macular hemorrhages includes size, pathology, thickness, age and duration, retinal layers affected, and foveal involvement of the bleeding. It will help clinicians in compiling most information relevant to set up the treatment strategy. Furthermore, it facilitates to set up study designs to compare different therapeutic approaches and their efficacy and to evaluate present or new treatment regimes.

References

1. Bopp S. [Subretinal hemorrhage. Natural course and staging]. Ophthalmologe. 2012;109(7):635–43.
2. Hohn F, Mirshahi A, Hattenbach LO. [Combined intravitreal injection of bevacizumab and SF6 gas for treatment of submacular hemorrhage secondary to age-related macular degeneration]. Ophthalmologe. 2010;107(4):328–32.
3. Nakamura H, Hayakawa K, Sawaguchi S, Gaja T, Nagamine N, Medoruma K. Visual outcome after vitreous, sub-internal limiting membrane, and/or submacular hemorrhage removal associated with ruptured retinal arterial macroaneurysms. Graefes Arch Clin Exp Ophthalmol. 2008;246(5):661–9.
4. Agostini HT, Bopp S, Feltgen N. [Prognosis and treatment of macular bleeding in neovascular age-related macular degeneration]. Ophthalmologe. 2017;114(5):476–80.
5. Avery RL, Fekrat S, Hawkins BS, Bressler NM. Natural history of subfoveal subretinal hemorrhage in age-related macular degeneration. Retina. 1996;16(3):183–9.
6. Scupola A, Coscas G, Soubrane G, Balestrazzi E. Natural history of macular subretinal hemorrhage in age-related macular degeneration. Ophthalmologica. 1999;213(2):97–102.
7. Freund KB, Zweifel SA, Engelbert M. Do we need a new classification for choroidal neovascularization in age-related macular degeneration? Retina. 2010;30(9):1333–49.
8. Glatt H, Machemer R. Experimental subretinal hemorrhage in rabbits. Am J Ophthalmol. 1982;94(6):762–73.
9. Stanescu-Segall D, Balta F, Jackson TL. Submacular hemorrhage in neovascular age-related macular degeneration: a synthesis of the literature. Surv Ophthalmol. 2016;61(1):18–32.
10. Dimopoulos S, Leitritz MA, Ziemssen F, Voykov B, Bartz-Schmidt KU, Gelisken F. Submacular predominantly hemorrhagic choroidal neovascularization: resolution of bleedings under anti-VEGF therapy. Clin Ophthalmol. 2015;9:1537–41.
11. Fassbender JM, Sherman MP, Barr CC, Schaal S. Tissue plasminogen activator for subfoveal hemorrhage due to age-related macular degeneration: comparison of 3 treatment modalities. Retina. 2016;36(10):1860–5.
12. De Maeyer K, Van Ginderdeuren R, Postelmans L, Stalmans P, Van Cealster J. Sub-inner limiting membrane haemorrhage: causes and treatment with vitrectomy. Br J Ophthalmol. 2007;91(7):869–72.
13. Fang IM, Lin YC, Yang CH, Yang CM, Chen MS. Effects of intravitreal gas with or without tissue plasminogen activator on submacular haemorrhage in age-related macular degeneration. Eye (Lond). 2009;23(2):397–406.
14. Chang W, Garg SJ, Maturi R, Hsu J, Sivalingam A, Gupta SA, et al. Management of thick submacular hemorrhage with subretinal tissue plasminogen activator and pneumatic displacement for age-related macular degeneration. Am J Ophthalmol. 2014;157(6):1250–7.
15. Stopa M, Kociecki J. [Macular translocation with 360 retinectomy for submacular hemorrhage in age related macular degeneration]. Klin Oczna. 2009;111(1–3):50–5.
16. Fine HF, Iranmanesh R, Del Priore LV, Barile GR, Chang LK, Chang S, et al. Surgical outcomes after massive subretinal hemorrhage secondary to age-related macular degeneration. Retina. 2010;30(10):1588–94.
17. Hochman MA, Seery CM, Zarbin MA. Pathophysiology and management of subretinal hemorrhage. Surv Ophthalmol. 1997;42(3):195–213.

18. Gaudreault J, Fei D, Beyer JC, Ryan A, Rangell L, Shiu V, et al. Pharmacokinetics and retinal distribution of ranibizumab, a humanized antibody fragment directed against VEGF-A, following intravitreal administration in rabbits. Retina. 2007;27(9):1260–6.
19. Sacu S, Stifter E, Vecsei-Marlovits PV, Michels S, Schutze C, Prunte C, et al. Management of extensive subfoveal haemorrhage secondary to neovascular age-related macular degeneration. Eye (Lond). 2009;23(6):1404–10.

Subretinal Co-application of rtPA and Bevacizumab for Neovascular AMD with Submacular Hemorrhage

4

Jost Hillenkamp

Introduction

Submacular hemorrhage (SMH) is not an unusual cause of acute central visual loss, particularly in the elderly. The most common cause is neovascular age-related macular degeneration (AMD). Without treatment, the long-term prognosis is usually poor because the underlying choroidal neovascularization (CNV) lesion progresses and the resolution of SMH is associated with the formation of a macular scar [1]. Invasive subretinal operations with removal of clotted submacular blood with or without CNV extraction have been abandoned because of poor functional outcome [2, 3]. In the early 1990s, recombinant tissue plasminogen activator (rtPA) was introduced to facilitate clot liquefaction in order to alleviate the trauma of subretinal manipulation. Functional improvement was reported in up to 60–80% patients, but still postoperative visual acuity was less than 20/200 in most cases [4]. With the aim to avoid surgical manipulation of the macular retina altogether, the displacement of SMH by intravitreal injection of rtPA and gas was proposed. According to several case series with this approach, SMH is successfully displaced in 60–100% of patients [5–7]. However, because of the size of the molecule, it is unclear whether or not intravitreally injected rtPA penetrates the retina to reach a subretinal clot [8–11]. Delivery of rtPA to the subretinal space may be ensured by subretinal injection [12–15]. In a case series of 11 patients reported by Haupert et al., pars plana vitrectomy (ppV) with subretinal injection of rtPA was shown to effectively clear SMH, but the procedure was associated with a 27% risk of hemorrhage recurrence [12]. Olivier et al. reported complete displacement of SMH in 25 of 28 patients with ppV with subretinal injection of rtPA, significant vision improvement in 17 patients, and minimal complications [13].

There are currently two principal surgical approaches which are applied with certain variations:

- Intravitreal injection of rtPA solution and a gas bubble [5–7]
- Subretinal injection of rtPA solution during pars plana vitrectomy (ppV) followed by an intravitreal gas bubble [12–16]

In the past, visual acuity often improved after successful displacement of SMH by rtPA and gas but then frequently deteriorated because of progression of the underlying CNV. Since the advent of anti-vascular endothelial growth factor (VEGF) pharmacotherapy, new aspects have been added to the management of neovascular AMD with SMH [17]. Due to the intriguing clinical results, a combined intraocular application of bevacizumab and rtPA seems to be a promising

J. Hillenkamp, MD
Department of Ophthalmology, University Hospital Würzburg, Würzburg, Germany

L.-O. Hattenbach (ed.), *Management of Macular Hemorrhage*,
https://doi.org/10.1007/978-3-319-65877-3_4

treatment for AMD with SMH. While an early application of rtPA can help to prevent an early toxic effect of SMH by effective displacement [12–14], the equally early application of anti-VEGF agents could potentially prevent CNV progression or recurrence.

Subretinal Co-application of rtPA and Bevacizumab: Surgical Technique

We developed a surgical technique for the subretinal co-application of rtPA and bevacizumab. Patients with submacular hemorrhage undergo a standard 20 gauge or 23 gauge three-port vitrectomy with induction of posterior hyaloid detachment if not already present, subretinal injection of 10–20 μg rtPA (Actilyse®, Boehringer Ingelheim, Germany) dissolved in 0.05–0.1 mL BSS followed by subretinal injection of 1.25 mg bevacizumab (Avastin®, Roche, Basel, Switzerland) dissolved in 0.05 mL BSS through a 41 gauge subretinal flexible cannula (D.O.R.C., Zuidland, The Netherlands), and fluid-gas exchange with 20% SF6 gas to a complete intravitreal fill. Subretinal injection is applied in areas of visibly subretinal but not sub-retinal pigment epithelium (RPE) hemorrhage in order to avoid the puncture of a pigment epithelial detachment (PED) and consecutive RPE-rip. Subretinal flexible cannulas are commercially available in 20-gauge or 23 gauge size. Fluid should be injected slowly into the subretinal space in order to avoid foveal rupture. We use two different insulin syringes for the rtPA and bevacizumab solutions which are injected consecutively. Phakic patients should undergo concomitant standard small-incision cataract surgery. Postoperatively, patients are instructed to keep a prone position for at least 1 day [15, 16].

Clinical Outcome

We reported on the short-term and long-term results of ppV with subretinal co-application of rtPA and bevacizumab followed by intravitreal fluid-gas exchange in a consecutive case series of 41 eyes [15, 16]. Postoperatively, all patients received at least two intravitreal injections of either bevacizumab or ranibizumab. The mean size of SMH was 4.5 disc diameters (range 1.5–12). Complete displacement of SMH was achieved in 35 of 41 eyes. Large and prominent SMH which extended beyond the temporal vascular arcades were successfully displaced in 6 of 8 eyes (Fig. 4.1). We observed recurrent SMH in 8 eyes at a mean of 9.1 months (range 2–19) after the initial operation. Systemic anticoagulation appears to be a risk factor as 6 of 8 patients with recurrent SMH were anticoagulated or had thrombocytopenia [15, 16]. In case of recurrent SMH, the same operation can be repeated, but the visual prognosis is usually poor.

During the first 12 months after the operation, a mean of 4.5 (range 2–9) intravitreal bevacizumab or ranibizumab injections were applied. At the time our reinjection scheme was based primarily on visual function. Short-term (3 months postop) mean logMAR best-corrected visual acuity (BCVA) improved from preop 1.7 (range 3.0–0.5) to 0.8 (range 1.6–0.2). Twelve eyes reached reading ability (≤logMAR 0.4), and 29 eyes reached ambulatory visual acuity (≤logMAR 1.6). Long-term (mean 17 months, range 12–32, $n = 26$) mean BCVA had worsened to logMAR 0.9 (range 1.6–0.1). As compared to the initial functional improvement, BCVA had worsened in 12 of 26 eyes (Fig. 4.2). The results show that medium-sized but also larger SMH can be effectively displaced from the fovea [15, 16].

In accordance with reports of anti-VEGF injection schemes for neovascular AMD without SMH [18, 19], our results suggest that a predominantly function-driven postoperative anti-VEGF re-treatment concept puts the initial functional improvement at a severe risk [15, 16]. It appears that in neovascular AMD, following initiation of anti-VEGF treatment, morphological changes precede functional changes as indicators of recurrence [20]. Because recurrent functional loss is less than fully reversible, an improved strict re-treatment regimen which prioritizes optical coherence tomography (OCT)-based morphological criteria over functional criteria with

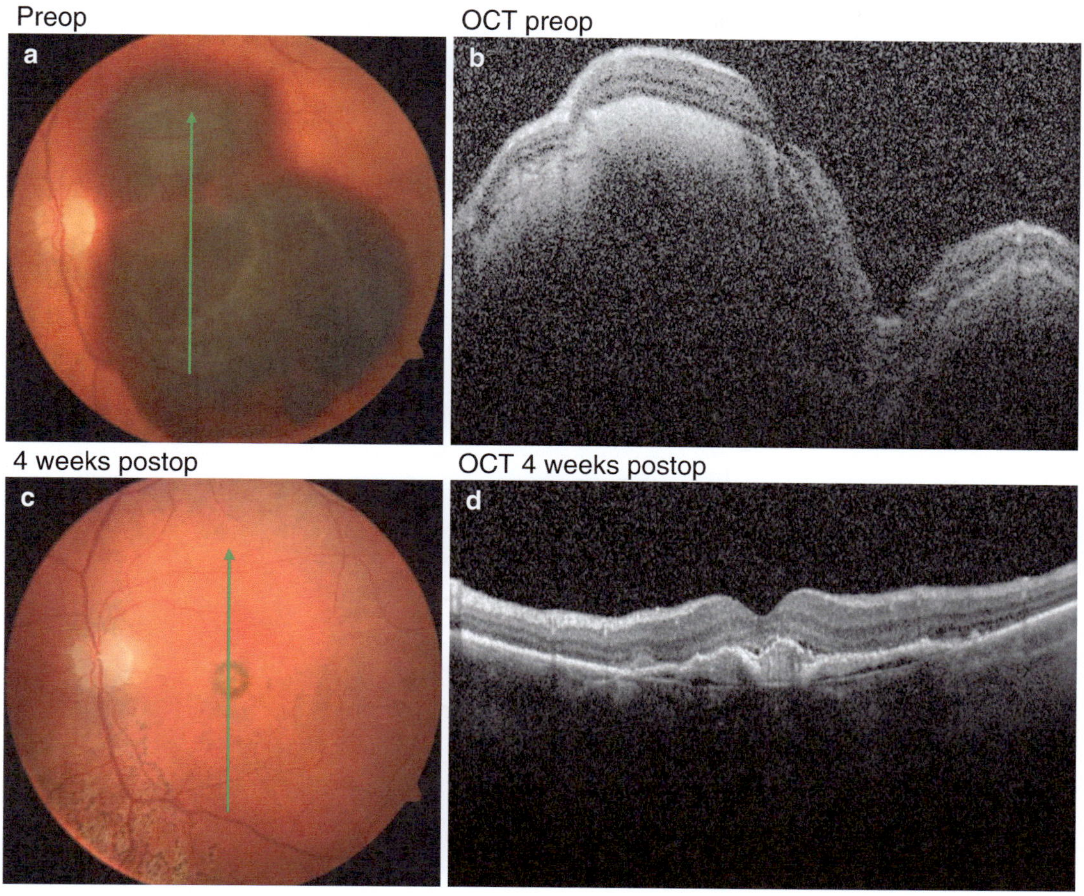

Fig. 4.1 Representative fundus photographs preop and 4 weeks post-op demonstrating complete displacement of large SMH extending beyond the vascular arcades. Optical coherence tomography (OCT) showed SMH preop and CNV post-op

early re-treatment when any sub- or intraretinal edema persists may lead to better long-term functional results [20, 21].

Of those patients with rather poor postoperative visual acuity, most felt a subjective benefit of the operation because of improvement of the central visual field after successful hemorrhage displacement.

In 24 of 25 phakic eyes, improvement of BCVA may have been caused to some degree by concomitant cataract surgery. Systematic preoperative cataract grading was not performed; however, the contribution of cataract surgery to the overall change of BCVA was probably small because the degree of lens opacity was described as mild in all phakic patients. Intraoperative complications occurred rarely and mainly in the early phase during our learning curve [15, 16]. We recommend preoperative OCT imaging to localize RPE detachment in order to avoid inadvertent puncture of the RPE with subsequent RPE-rip. Subretinal injection should be performed slowly with a maximal total volume of 0.1 mL in order to avoid rupture of retinal tissue at the fovea, the point of least mechanical resistance.

Eighteen patients in our study were on anticoagulation treatment, and two patients had a coagulation disorder. Our results suggest that anticoagulation is probably a risk factor for the development and recurrence of SMH. Seven of 8 SMH recurrences occurred in patients either with systemic anticoagulation or thrombocytopenia [15, 16]. The risk of recurrence may be reduced by early CNV regression induced by the simultaneous application of bevacizumab. Principally, the initial operation can be repeated in case of SMH recurrence. In our study recurrent SMH was successfully displaced in five of six eyes; however, functional improvement was limited [15, 16]. Since recurrences occurred during an extended period after surgery, we recommend a strict postoperative anti-VEGF re-treatment regimen and, if possible, discontinuation of systemic anticoagulation, especially in only-eye situations.

Intraoperative complications were rare. Most complications can be avoided by applying appropriate caution during surgery. In our case series, we had one case of intraoperative RPE-rip, one case of intraoperative foveal rupture during subretinal injection, and one case of postoperative rhegmatogenous retinal detachment [15, 16].

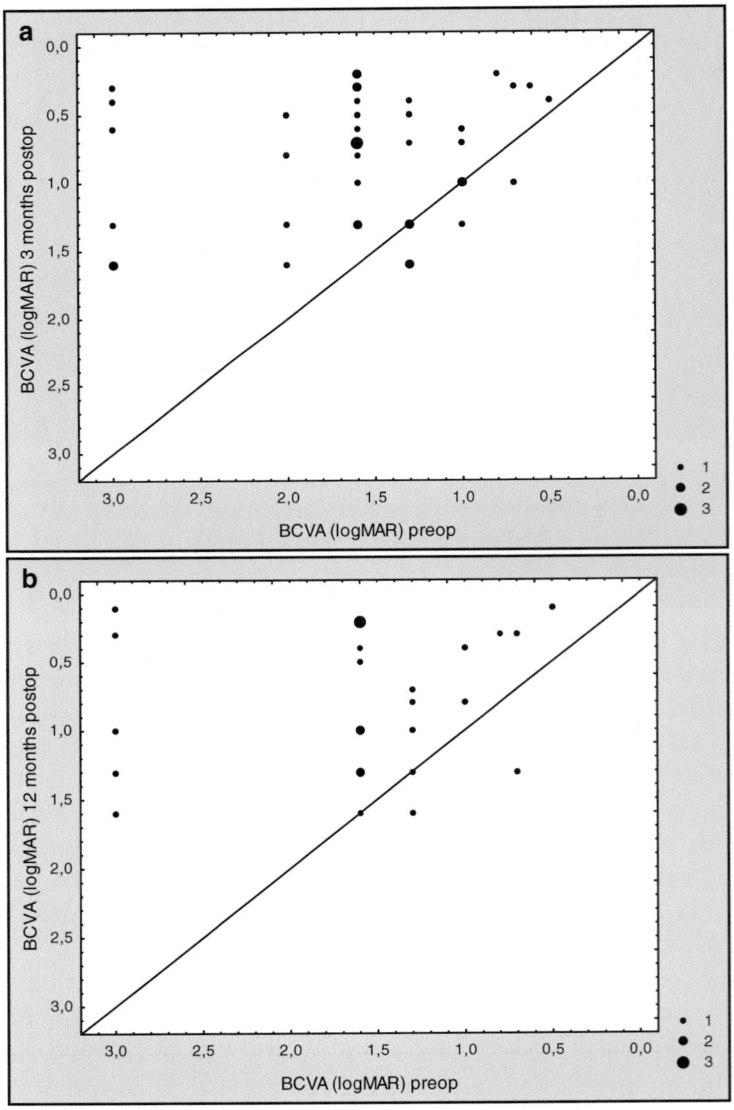

Fig. 4.2 Scatterplots comparing pre- and postoperative BCVA (logMAR) at 3 months follow-up (**a**), 12 months follow-up (**b**), final follow-up (mean 17 months, range 12–32) (**c**), and comparing BCVA at 3 months post-op with final follow-up (**d**)

Fig. 4.2 (continued)

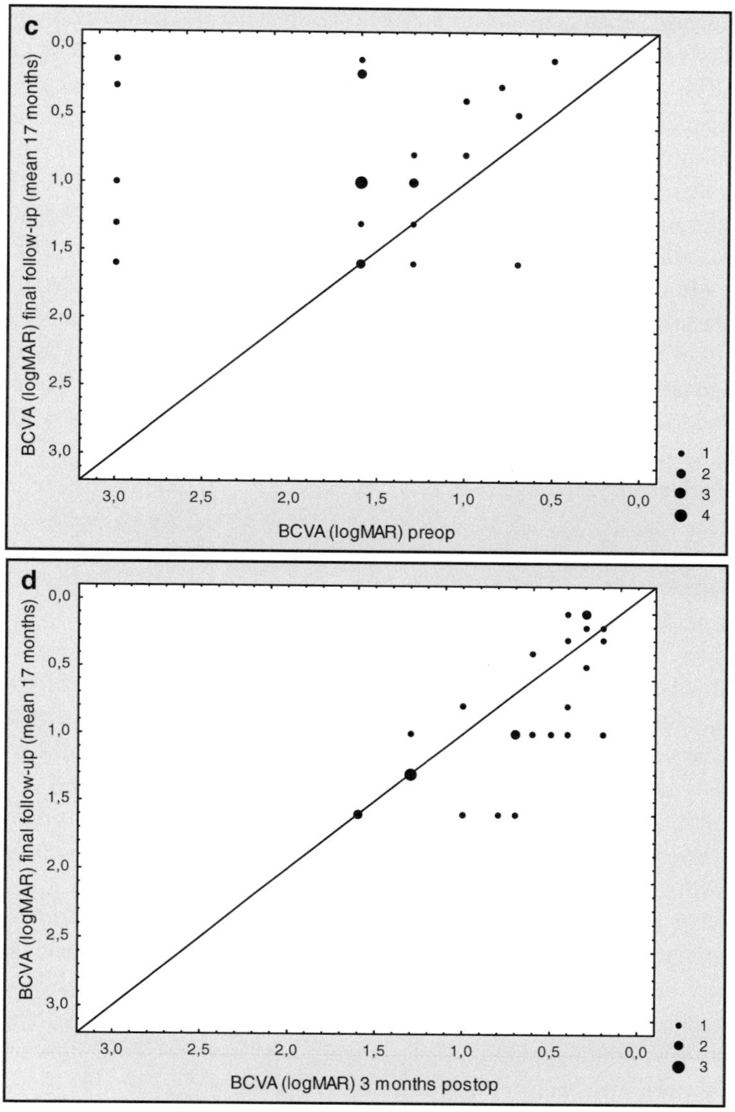

Compatibility of rtPA and Bevacizumab: Experimental Studies

Background

While the functional and anatomical results of subretinal co-application of rtPA and bevacizumab are promising [15, 16], it has been unclear whether or not co-applied rtPA and bevacizumab are compatible. rtPA is a serine protease with its catalytic activity around the B chain (light chain). The serine protease family possesses a triad characteristically formed of a serine, a histidine, and an aspartate. The hydroxyl group of the serine plays a role in the nucleophile and attacks the carbonyl peptide bond. rtPA cleaves after the arginine, but other amino acids determine the specificity of rtPA. The main substrate of rtPA is plasminogen which cleaves into active plasmin. Plasmin then degrades the fibrin matrix which constitutes blood clots. However, other proteins such as hepatocyte growth factor [22] or platelet-derived growth factor [23] are also cleaved by rtPA. Hence, it is uncertain whether in co-application either rtPA itself, or rtPA-generated plasmin, or other undetermined proteases activated during fibrinolysis of a subretinal blood clot may cleave and thereby functionally inactivate the antibody bevacizumab.

In several experimental studies, we investigated the compatibility of rtPA and bevacizumab as well as of plasmin and bevacizumab in an in vitro model of their intraoperative co-application as a treatment of acute SMH in neovascular AMD, assessing potential cleavage as well as anti-angiogenic functionality of bevacizumab.

Interaction of rtPA, Plasmin, and Bevacizumab

In all experiments we used mixing ratios of rtPA and bevacizumab similar to those during surgery. The compatibility of plasmin and bevacizumab was tested using plasmin derived from human plasma [24]. The possible interaction of either rtPA or plasmin and bevacizumab was analyzed with electrophoresis. The electrophoresis gels were stained with coomassie and silver, photographed, using a Bio-Image system, and the density and size of the electrophoresis bands were analyzed using a special software [24].

We found no additional bands when rtPA and bevacizumab were co-applied. As compared to coomassie staining, silver staining revealed additional bands. Also with silver staining, there were no additional bands when rtPA and bevacizumab were co-applied. The plasmin bands were not detected in the mixtures. As compared to the coomassie staining, silver staining revealed additional bands. All bevacizumab bands are also seen when bevacizumab was co-applied with either rtPA or plasmin.

Anti-VEGF Effectivity of Bevacizumab

We used a porcine RPE cell culture model to quantify the anti-angiogenic effectivity of bevacizumab co-applied with either rtPA or plasmin or plasmin together with human blood. Confluent cultured RPE cells release VEGF into the culture medium [25]. We added bevacizumab and rtPA or plasmin and quantified the anti-VEGF effectivity of bevacizumab with ELISA. To simulate the intraoperative situation and to test whether bevacizumab remains effective together with rtPA in the presence of blood, we incubated the culture medium with bevacizumab, rtPA, and human blood and quantified VEGF in the medium with ELISA. We detected virtually no VEGF in the culture medium following co-incubation of bevacizumab with either rtPA or plasmin. The anti-VEGF effectivity of bevacizumab was also not compromised in the presence of rtPA and human blood (Fig. 4.3).

Clinical Significance of the Compatibility of Bevacizumab and rtPA

Our results demonstrate that in co-application of bevacizumab and rtPA during surgery:

- Bevacizumab is not cleaved by either rtPA or rtPA-generated plasmin
- Anti-VEGF effectivity of bevacizumab remains uncompromised when co-applied with rtPA with or without plasmin or human blood

In electrophoresis we have used coomassie staining and additionally silver staining as a second method to confirm the findings and to detect additional bands not stained by coomassie. With both stains the band patterns clearly show that no additional bands appear when bevacizumab is co-incubated with either rtPA or plasmin; hence, bevacizumab remains structurally intact.

Our results confirm the results of Faure et al. who also found an absence of cleavage of bevacizumab by rtPA in electrophoresis [26]. However, our study [24] adds important new findings because we show that besides rtPA also rtPA-generated active plasmin does not cleave

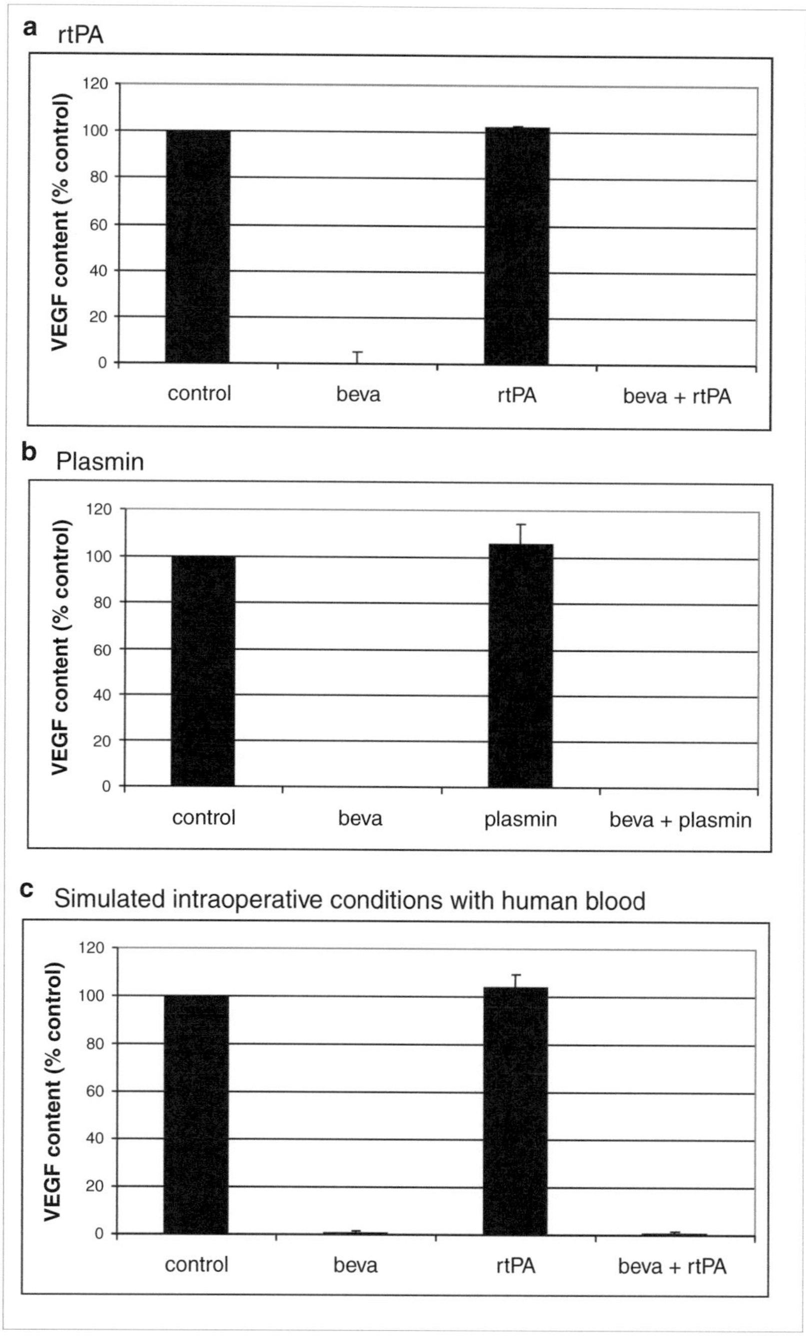

Fig. 4.3 Bevacizumab functionality. Ability of bevacizumab to impair the recognition of VEGF by VEGF ELISA in the presence of (**a**) rtPA, (**b**) plasmin, and (**c**) human blood clot dissolved by rtPA in simulated intraoperative conditions. VEGF content is depicted as % of control. The ability of bevacizumab to inhibit VEGF is not altered in either experimental setting. *Beva* bevacizumab. Error bars depict standard deviation

bevacizumab. We additionally used silver stain, a more sensitive staining method, to confirm the results. Furthermore, electrophoresis alone does not prove the therapeutic compatibility of the two agents. Electrophoresis itself fragments bevacizumab which implies that bevacizumab fragments generated by rtPA would not be identified as such if they are of the same molecular weight as the fragments generated by electrophoresis. Even cleaved bevacizumab could still be functional as long as the cleavage does not interfere with VEGF binding. Hence, in order to reliably determine the functionality of bevacizumab co-applied with rtPA, we quantified binding of VEGF by bevacizumab when co-incubated with rtPA or plasmin. Furthermore, other possible mechanisms of impairment of the anti-angiogenic effect of bevacizumab when injected into the area of SMH in patients include a possible interaction with blood as (1) platelets have been shown to take up bevacizumab [27] and (2) bevacizumab could be cleaved and functionally inactivated by undetermined proteases activated during fibrinolysis of the subretinal blood clot. We therefore used an in vitro model of the intraoperative situation with rtPA incubated with clotted human blood followed by a test of the effect of the resulting liquid on the functionality of bevacizumab. The amount of human blood used in the ELISA experiments was greater than the calculated volumes of SMH. However, an excess amount of blood ascertains that all bevacizumab molecules in the solution would be saturated with undetermined proteolytic enzymes potentially activated during fibrinolysis. Our ELISA experiments clearly show that neither rtPA, plasmin, nor proteases activated during fibrinolysis of a subretinal blood clot functionally inactivate bevacizumab [24].

Intravitreal vs. Subretinal Application of rtPA and Bevacizumab

Our experimental results are relevant to the clinical management of acute SMH in neovascular AMD. Intravitreal [18, 19] and subretinal [14–16] co-application of rtPA and bevacizumab have been reported. Whether intravitreal or subretinal application of rtPA combined with an intravitreal gas bubble is the better approach to displace SMH is the subject of an ongoing debate. So far, there is no adequately designed prospective randomized clinical trial to investigate this open question. In a previous retrospective consecutive case series, we compared ppV with either intravitreal or subretinal injection of rtPA and fluid-gas exchange. We found that subretinal injection of rtPA was more effective in terms of complete displacement of SMH. Functional improvement in the majority of our patients suggested the absence of direct retinal toxicity of subretinally applied rtPA [14]. Both rtPA and bevacizumab are relatively large molecules which exceed the experimentally determined molecular exclusion limit of human retina [10]. Bevacizumab has been shown to traverse healthy retina [11], but it probably does so only at a slow rate because of its size [10]. It is unclear whether intravitreally injected rtPA penetrates the retina as rtPA injected into the vitreous of rabbits failed to pass through healthy retina [8]. On the other hand, molecules with similar molecular weight (e.g., albumin) have been shown to penetrate the diseased retina [9]. A subretinal blood clot may hamper transretinal diffusion, and following intravitreal injection, both agents may not reach the subretinal space and the underlying CNV at a sufficient concentration. However, while the intravitreal application of rtPA and bevacizumab may suffice to produce a therapeutic response [18, 19], subretinal application [14–16] ensures direct liquefaction of clotted subretinal blood by rtPA and the delivery of bevacizumab directly at the site of the CNV which may enhance its effect. Our experimental finding of the absence of functional inactivation of bevacizumab in the presence of rtPA and blood is clinically relevant as in intravitreal, and perhaps even more so in subretinal co-application, not only the two drugs possibly interact but also bevacizumab and proteolytic enzymes released from the liquefied blood clot.

Experimental studies to test the compatibility of rtPA, plasmin, and ranibizumab, or aflibercept are currently underway.

References

1. Avery RL, Fekrat S, Hawkins BS, et al. Natural history of subfoveal hemorrhage in age-related macular degeneration. Retina. 1996;16:183–9.
2. Vander JF, Federman JL, Greven C, Slusher MM, Gabel VP. Surgical removal of massive subretinal hemorrhage associated with age-related macular degeneration. Ophthalmology. 1991;98:23–7.
3. Bressler NM, Bressler SB, Childs AL et al., for Submacular Surgery Trials (SST) Research Group. Surgery for hemorrhagic choroidal neovascular lesions of age-related macular degeneration: ophthalmic findings: SST report No. 13. Ophthalmology. 2004;111:1993–2006.

4. Lewis H. Intraoperative fibrinolysis of submacular hemorrhage with tissue plasminogen activator and surgical drainage. Am J Ophthalmol. 1994;118:559–68.
5. Chen CY, Hooper C, Chiu D, Chamberlain M, Karia N, Heriot WJ. Management of submacular hemorrhage with intravitreal injection of tissue plasminogen activator and expansile gas. Retina. 2007;27:321–8.
6. Hesse L, Schmidt J, Kroll P. Management of acute submacular hemorrhage using recombinant tissue plasminogen activator and gas. Graefes Arch Clin Exp Ophthalmol. 1999;237:273–7.
7. Handwerger BA, Blodi BA, Chandra SR, Olsen TW, Stevens TS. Treatment of submacular hemorrhage with low-dose intravitreal tissue plasminogen activator injection and pneumatic displacement. Arch Ophthalmol. 2001;119:28–32.
8. Kamei M, Misono K, Lewis H. A study of the ability of tissue plasminogen activator to diffuse into the subretinal space after intravitreal injection in rabbits. Am J Ophthalmol. 1999;128:739–46.
9. Takeuchi A, Kricorian G, Yao XY, et al. The rate and source of albumin entry into saline-filled experimental retinal detachments. Invest Ophthalmol Vis Sci. 1994;35:3792–598.
10. Jackson TL, Antcliff RJ, Hillenkamp J, Marshall J. Human retinal molecular weight exclusion limit and estimate of species variation. Invest Ophthalmol Vis Sci. 2003;44:2141–6.
11. Heiduschka P, Fietz H, Hofmeister S, et al. Penetration of bevacizumab through the retina after intravitreal injection in the monkey. Invest Ophthalmol Vis Sci. 2007;48:2814–23.
12. Haupert CL, BW MC II, Jaffe GJ. Pars plana vitrectomy, subretinal injection of tissue plasminogen activator, and fluid-gas exchange for displacement of thick submacular hemorrhage in age-related macular degeneration. Am J Ophthalmol. 2001;131:208–15.
13. Olivier S, Chow DR, Packo KH. Subretinal recombinant tissue plasminogen activator injection and pneumatic displacement of thick submacular hemorrhage in age-related macular degeneration. Ophthalmology. 2004;111:1201–8.
14. Hillenkamp J, Surguch V, Framme C, Gabel VP, Sachs HG. Management of submacular hemorrhage with intravitreal versus subretinal injection of recombinant tissue plasminogen activator. Graefes Arch Clin Exp Ophthalmol. 2010;248:5–11.
15. Treumer F, Klatt C, Roider J, Hillenkamp J. Subretinal co-application of recombinant tissue plasminogen activator and bevacizumab for neovascular age-related macular degeneration with submacular hemorrhage. Br J Ophthalmol. 2010;94:48–53.
16. Treumer F, Roider J, Hillenkamp J. Long-term outcome of subretinal co-application of rtPA and bevacizumab followed by repeated intravitreal anti-VEGF injections for neovascular AMD with submacular hemorrhage. Br J Ophthalmol. 2012;96:708–13.
17. Schouten JS, La Heij EC, Webers CA, et al. A systematic review on the effect of bevacizumab in exudative age-related macular degeneration. Graefes Arch Clin Exp Ophthalmol. 2009;247:1–11.
18. Heimes B, Lommatzsch A, Zeimer M, Gutfleisch M, Spital G, Dietzel M, Pauleikhoff D. Long-term visual course after anti-VEGF therapy for exudative AMD in clinical practice evaluation of the German reinjection scheme. Graefes Arch Clin Exp Ophthalmol. 2010;249:639–44.
19. Dadgostar H, Ventura AA, Chung JY, Sharma S, Kaiser PK. Evaluation of injection frequency and visual acuity outcomes for ranibizumab monotherapy in exudative age-related macular degeneration. Ophthalmology. 2009;116:1740–7.
20. Gerding H, Loukopoulos V, Riese J, Hefner L, Timmermann M. Results of flexible ranibizumab treatment in age-related macular degeneration and search for parameters with impact on outcome. Graefes Arch Clin Exp Ophthalmol. 2011;249:653–62.
21. Pauleikhoff D, Kirchhof B. Retreatment criteria in anti-VEGF therapy of exudative AMD: critical analysis of present regimes and new morphological definition of "lesion activity". Graefes Arch Clin Exp Ophthalmol. 2011;249:631–2.
22. Mars WM, Zarnegar R, Michalopoulos GK. Activation of hepatocyte growth factor by the plasminogen activators uPA and tPA. Am J Pathol. 1993;143:949–858.
23. Su EJ, Fredriksson L, Geyer M, et al. Activation of PDGF-CC by tissue plasminogen activator impairs blood-brain barrier integrity during ischemic stroke. Nat Med. 2008;14:731–7.
24. Klettner A, Puls S, Treumer F, Roider J, Hillenkamp J. Compatibility of recombinant tissue plasminogen activator (rtPA) and bevacizumab co-applied for neovascular age-related macular degeneration with submacular hemorrhage. Arch Ophthalmol. 2012;130:875–81.
25. Klettner A, Roider J. Comparison of bevacizumab, ranibizumab, and pegaptanib in vitro: efficiency and possible additional pathways. Invest Ophthalmol Vis Sci. 2008;49:4523–7.
26. Faure C, Macrez R, Vivien D, Sahel JA, Bonnel S. Interaction study between rtPA and bevacizumab. Br J Ophthalmol. 2011;95:743–4.
27. Verheul HM, Lolkema MP, Qian DZ, et al. Platelets take up the monoclonal antibody bevacizumab. Clin Cancer Res. 2007;13:5341–7.

Minimally Invasive Surgical Treatment of Macular Hemorrhages

5

Lars-Olof Hattenbach

Introduction

Macular hemorrhages secondary to retinal macroaneurysms or choroidal neovascularization (CNV) associated with age-related macular degeneration (ARMD) or myopia can cause sudden visual loss. Although such patients occasionally may have spontaneous improvement in visual acuity, the overall prognosis of untreated submacular hemorrhage is poor [1–5]. Experimental studies have demonstrated that irreversible retinal damage occurs as early as 24 h after the onset of hemorrhage [6, 7]. In a clinical study, the eyes with subfoveal hemorrhage secondary to ARMD exhibited a loss of three or more lines of visual acuity from baseline in 48% of all cases after a follow-up of 6 months. Other researchers found that patients with subretinal hemorrhage due to ARMD had a considerable decrease in visual acuity over time, with an average visual acuity of 20/1700 at the final follow-up visit. Interestingly, there was no direct association between visual outcome and thickness or size of the hemorrhage.

Attempts to treat massive submacular hemorrhage with vitreoretinal surgery to remove the subretinal blood clot often yield disappointing results [8–11]. From the current data, surgical intervention may only be recommended in selected cases [12, 13]. Moreover, in view of a high rate of intraoperative and postoperative complications, concern about a surgical approach is particularly pertinent for patients with small areas of subretinal blood.

Recognition of the damaging effects of subretinal blood has stimulated interest in minimally invasive strategies to improve patients' visual recovery. In 1996, Heriot reported on the management of submacular hemorrhage with intravitreally injected recombinant tissue plasminogen activator (rt-PA) and pneumatic displacement as an alternative to vitrectomy and surgical drainage [14]. The use of fibrinolytic agents appears to be an ideal approach to a minimally invasive treatment of subretinal hemorrhage [15–20]. Intravitreally injected rt-PA can migrate across the retina, thereby facilitating the dissolution of subretinal blood. In experimental studies, subretinal blood clots disappeared within 24 h after intravitreal injections of rt-PA in the rabbit, whereas there was no change in control eyes injected with saline solution [21]. Moreover, it has been demonstrated that albumin, a protein with a molecular weight similar to that of t-PA, is detectable in the subretinal space within 1 h, suggesting that rt-PA might not be exempt from traversing the retina [22]. Other investigators found a causal relationship between change of hemorrhage size and subretinal clot lysis induced by rt-PA in ARMD patients. They explained the diffusion of rt-PA across the retina by retinal microlesions secondary to subretinal blood clots [23].

L.-O. Hattenbach, M.D., F.E.B.O.
Department of Ophthalmology, Ludwigshafen Hospital, Ludwigshafen, Germany

L.-O. Hattenbach (ed.), *Management of Macular Hemorrhage*,
https://doi.org/10.1007/978-3-319-65877-3_5

The encouraging initial experience reported by Heriot has been further substantiated by the findings of other investigators. In this chapter, we present the results from our own study which is among the largest case series investigating the treatment of subretinal hemorrhage with intravitreal rt-PA and gas injection and discuss the results from concurrent trials. However, although most of these early studies demonstrated that intravitreal injection of rt-PA and gas is effective in displacing thick submacular blood and facilitating visual improvement, final visual outcomes were limited by the progression of the underlying macular disease because there was no effective therapy for the management of choroidal neovascularization (CNV).

More recent minimally invasive treatment approaches used combined small-gauge core vitrectomy, pneumatic displacement, rt-PA-induced fibrinolysis, and intravitreal anti-VEGF agents. To date, there is much evidence that combined treatments targeting at clot lysis, mechanical displacement, and inhibition of neovascularization have the potential to yield excellent results, thereby providing a minimally invasive alternative to extensive vitreoretinal surgery.

Intravitreal Injection of rt-PA and Hexafluoride

Methods and Procedure

The procedure is performed under topical anesthesia with 2% lidocaine. Prior to injection, betadine is applied to the lids and periorbita, and the eye is irrigated with sterile saline. This may be followed by neomycin sulfate drops. Fifty micrograms of commercial rt-PA solution (Actilyse, Boehringer, Ingelheim, Germany) in a volume of 50 μL is drawn in a tuberculin syringe and injected into the midvitreous cavity through a 30-gauge needle. After an aqueous tap to reduce intraocular pressure, 0.5 mL of 100% sulfur hexafluoride gas is injected into the vitreous cavity. Both injections are administered via the pars plana in the superotemporal or superonasal quadrant, 3 mm posterior to the limbus in pseudophakic patients and 3.5 mm posterior to the limbus in phakic patients. Patients are then instructed to maintain prone positioning for 72 h. Whenever blood displacement from under the fovea is not complete, prone positioning may be continued for 24–48 h.

In a prospective case series of 43 consecutive eyes (42 patients), we investigated the efficacy and safety of treating submacular hemorrhages secondary to age-related macular degeneration (ARMD) with intravitreal rt-PA and expansile gas under various conditions [24]. The objective of this investigation was to determine the efficacy and safety of this minimally invasive procedure and the predictive value of various clinical baseline characteristics with regard to visual outcome. Moreover, since there was no consensus about indication criteria or the ideal timing after the onset of subretinal hemorrhage, we attempted to determine the usefulness of this approach in the management of small subfoveal hemorrhages. All patients had acute ($\leq$28 days) submacular hemorrhage secondary to ARMD centered in or close to the fovea and reading vision in the affected eye prior to the onset of hemorrhage. Patients were excluded whenever vitreous hemorrhage was present at the initial examination. Primary outcome measures were best and final postoperative visual acuity and degree of blood displacement. Changes in visual acuity were defined as improvement, i.e., increase of two or more Snellen visual acuity lines; stable, i.e., within <2 lines from baseline visual acuity; and worse, i.e., loss of two or more Snellen visual acuity lines. The degree of blood displacement was measured ophthalmoscopically after completion of prone positioning and graded as complete, i.e., $\geq$1 disc area from the center of the fovea, partial, or no displacement. Presenting characteristics such as age, gender, initial visual acuity, duration of subretinal hemorrhage prior to treatment, and initial size of hemorrhage (disc diameters) were used to subdivide patients and to investigate their prognostic value. In all patients, complete bilateral ocular examinations were conducted, at the initial examination, 1–5 days after treatment and at 2–6-week intervals. In all cases, follow-up data were obtained over a minimum period of 4 months (range 4–18 months). The size of the subfoveal hemorrhage was measured in standardized Macular Photocoagulation Study (MPS) disc areas. The presence of a submacular neovascular lesion was confirmed by ophthalmoscopy and fluorescein angiography. All patients received intravitreal injections of rt-PA (50 μg) and sulfur hexafluoride (0.5 mL). Postoperative prone positioning was maintained for 24–72 h.

Outcome

Visual outcome was analyzed in relation to size and onset of hemorrhage, displacement of subretinal blood, and surgical complications. Best postoperative visual acuity compared with preoperative visual acuity was improved by two or more Snellen lines in 19 eyes (44%) and stable in 24 eyes (56%). Final visual acuity was improved two or more lines in 13 eyes (30%), stable in 26 (61%), and two or more lines worse in 4 eyes (9%). Best postoperative acuity was maintained for an average of 4.2 months, with a range of 0.5–12 months. After a mean follow-up time of 6 months, visual acuity was improved two or more lines in 30% of patients (Fig. 5.1). Best and final acuities ranged from counting fingers to 20/30. Twenty-one eyes (49%) achieved a best visual acuity better than 20/200, and 15 eyes (35%) maintained this level at the final visit. Four of these eyes (9%) attained a final visual acuity of 20/50 or better.

The findings of our study were supported by other investigators who observed a beneficial effect of intravitreally injected rt-PA and pneumatic displacement in submacular hemorrhage. Hassan et al. observed a complete displacement of submacular blood in 100% and a final visual improvement of two or more lines in 67% in the eyes with thick submacular hemorrhage ranging from 2 to 13 disc areas after treatment with intravitreal rt-PA [25]. Other researchers observed an improvement in visual acuity by two lines in 45.5% of the eyes after intravitreal injections of 50–100 μg of rt-PA and gas in the eyes with submacular hemorrhage secondary to ARMD [26].

We observed a complete displacement of blood from under the fovea in 81% (35 eyes) and partial displacement in 19% (8 eyes), indicating that blood displacement can be achieved in the majority of cases (Fig. 5.2). However, the observation that only 44% of all patients developed postoperative visual improvement supports evidence that functional outcome is limited by retinal damage associated with size and duration of subretinal blood clot formation. Overall, the size of subreti-

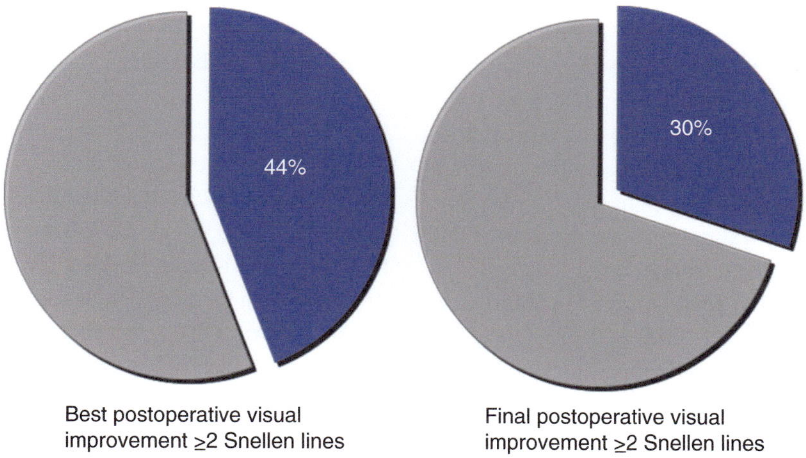

Fig. 5.1 Best postoperative visual acuity after injection of rt-PA and hexafluoride gas was improved by two or more Snellen lines in 44% and stable in 56% of all cases. Final visual acuity was improved two or more lines in 30%, stable in 61%, and two or more lines worse in 9%. Best postoperative acuity was maintained for an average of 4.2 months, with a range of 0.5–12 months

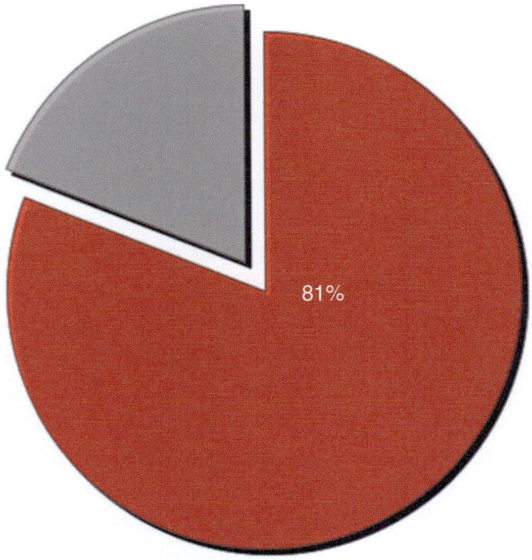

Fig. 5.2 After injection of rt-PA and hexafluoride gas, blood displacement can be achieved in the majority of cases. We observed a complete displacement of blood from under the fovea in 81% and partial displacement in 19% of cases

nal hemorrhage ranged from 1/4 to 30 disc areas (Fig. 5.3), with a mean duration of subretinal hemorrhage of 15.4 days, ranging from 2 to 28 days.

Safety

Overall, the intravitreal injection of rt-PA and gas appears to be a safe procedure. In our case series, we observed no major intraoperative or postoperative complications. Nine eyes (21%) developed recurrent hemorrhage which required repeat treatment, whereas breakthrough vitreous hemorrhage occurred in 7% of patients. Repeat treatment with rt-PA and gas was not associated with a higher risk of hemorrhage.

The potentially toxic effects of intravitreal rt-PA have long been discussed previously. We found no evidence of retinal or other intraocular toxic reactions to rt-PA at a dose of 50 µg used in our study, and this is consistent with the findings of other investigators who observed no signs of retinal toxicity. From the available data, there is much evidence that that retinal toxicity from intravitreally injected rt-PA is a dose-dependent problem. Hesse et al. reported exudative retinal detachment, RPE hyperpigmentation, and a marked reduction in the electroretinogram postoperatively in the eyes that received intravitreal rt-PA injections of 100 µg, but not in the eyes treated with 50 µg [23]. In an experimental study, Johnson et al. found no toxic reactions in rabbit eyes after injections of rt-PA at a dose of 25 µg, whereas one of four eyes injected with 50 µg showed localized loss of photoreceptor cells and severe retinal damage was seen at higher concentrations [27]. This was attributed to the L-arginine vehicle of the commercially available rt-PA solution. Hrach and coworkers observed fundus pigmentary alterations and a loss of photoreceptor elements in cat eyes receiving commercial rt-PA solution in doses greater than or equal to 50 µg [28]. However, the larger vitreous volume, greater vitreous liquefaction, and vascularized retina in human eyes may raise the threshold for toxicity and help explain the favorable results of clinical studies that used higher concentrations of rt-PA.

Despite the potential damaging effects, intravitreal rt-PA appears to be an important component for a successful minimally invasive pneumatic displacement of subretinal blood. Results from studies that attempted to treat subfoveal hemorrhage with intravitreal injections of gas alone indicate that this therapeutic approach is less effective and may only be useful in the eyes with a short treatment interval of several days [29].

Predictive Factors

One of the most striking findings of our study was the observation that a short duration of hemorrhage was associated with a better gain of lines of vision ($P = 0.0058$). Of those eyes with duration of hemorrhage ≤14 days, two thirds (67%) improved two or more Snellen lines to their best postoperative acuity, compared with one third (29%) of the eyes with duration of hemorrhage >14 days. By the end of the follow-up period, 43% of the eyes with duration of hemorrhage ≤14 days had gained two or more Snellen lines, whereas only 18% of the eyes with clots of longer duration showed a comparable outcome. In contrast, none of the eyes with a symptom to treatment interval >21 days showed an improvement

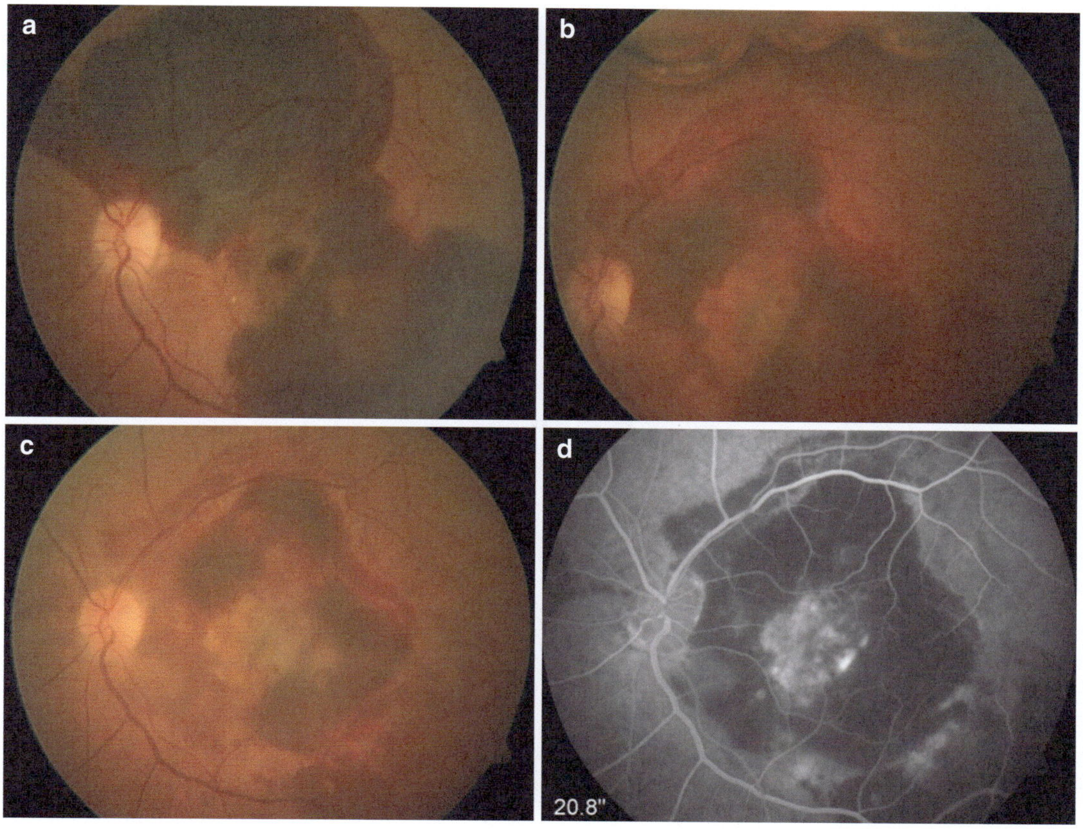

Fig. 5.3 (**a–d**) Fundus photographs of a patient with large subfoveal hemorrhage before (**a**), 1 day (**b**) and 1 week (**c**) after injection of rt-PA and hexafluoride, demonstrating an inferotemporal shift of subretinal blood after therapy. (**d**) Shows the postoperative fluorescein angiogram revealing subfoveal choroidal neovascularization

from initial to final postoperative visual acuity. It appears that duration of hemorrhage is a strong predictor of visual recovery after treatment with rt-PA and gas in subretinal hemorrhage.

In contrast to previous investigations, we included subjects with small submacular hemorrhages, i.e., ≤2 disc areas. It may be speculated that such eyes have a generally better prognosis. However, we found no direct relationship between hemorrhage size alone and better postoperative visual recovery, whereas subgroup analysis for only those patients with small hemorrhage size revealed that a short time (≤14 days) from onset of hemorrhage to treatment was associated with a better gain of lines of vision [30]. Among the eyes with duration of hemorrhage equal to or less than 14 days and hemorrhage size ≤2 disc areas, 78% were observed to improve two or more lines of vision after treatment. Only 25% of those eyes with hemorrhage size ≤2 disc areas and duration of hemorrhage >14 days improved two or more Snellen visual acuity lines (Fig. 5.4).

These findings highlight the potential for improved retinal survival and visual recovery after early minimally invasive therapeutic intervention with rt-PA and gas in the eyes with limited damage secondary to the formation of subretinal blood clots. Experimental studies identified clot retraction as a major cause of damage in subretinal hemorrhage, and there is much evidence that hemorrhage size and time from onset play a major role. By using different animal models, it has been demonstrated that photoreceptors degenerated in less than 24 h. Severe outer retinal degeneration occurred within 3–7 days in the rabbit retina and within 7–14 days in the cat retina [31].

Another preoperative factor found to have an effect on absolute final acuity was preoperative visual acuity which ranged from hand motions to 20/50. Of the 15 eyes with final visual acuity

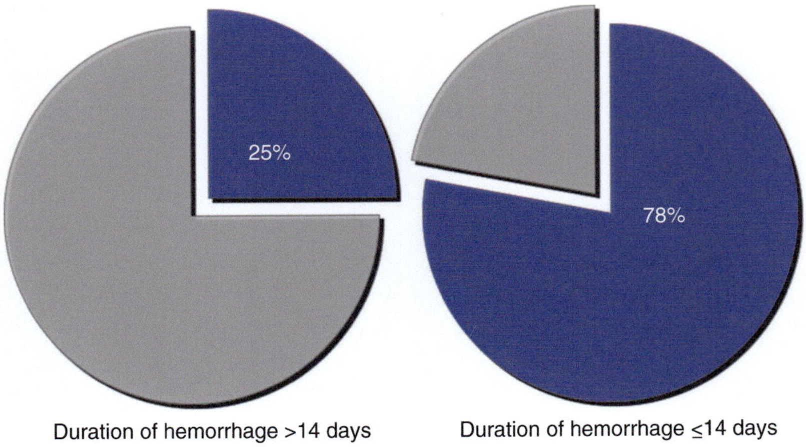

Fig. 5.4 Size and duration of hemorrhage are strong predictive factors of visual outcome after treatment with intravitreal rt-PA and hexafluoride gas. Subgroup analysis for only those patients with small hemorrhage size revealed that a short time to treatment, i.e., ≤14 days from onset of hemorrhage, was associated with a better gain of lines of vision. Among the eyes with duration of hemorrhage equal to or less than 14 days and hemorrhage size ≤2 disc areas, 78% were observed to improve two or more lines of vision after treatment, whereas only 25% of those eyes with hemorrhage size ≤2 disc areas and duration of hemorrhage >14 days showed a comparable outcome

equal to or better than 20/100, 8 (53%) had an initial visual acuity ≥20/100, whereas only 2 of 28 eyes (7%) with final acuity less than 20/100 had ≥20/100 initial vision (P = 0.0013). Better preoperative visual acuity (≥20/100) was not associated with a gain of lines (≥2 Snellen lines) of vision (P = 0.14, n.s.). Factors that had no significant effect on final visual outcome included patient age and gender [24].

Intravitreal Anti-VEGF Monotherapy and Combined Intravitreal Administration of Anti-VEGF Agents and Expansile Gas

To date, the intravitreal administration of anti-VEGF drugs is the standard of care in the management of choroidal neovascularization secondary to AMD [32–35]. However, the efficacy of intravitreal anti-VEGF monotherapy in the management of CNV associated with subretinal hemorrhage has not been subject to extensive investigations. Inclusion criteria of most studies investigating the efficacy and safety of intravitreal anti-VEGF drugs precluded a detailed analysis with regard to outcomes in subgroups of AMD patients with subretinal hemorrhage. However, available data suggest that choroidal neovascularization secondary to age-related macular degeneration associated with small subretinal hemorrhages may well be treated with anti-VEGF monotherapy [36–39].

With the advent of anti-VEGF agents, continued treatment of underlying choroidal neovascularization to prevent recurrent hemorrhage after successful displacement of submacular blood has become feasible. Furthermore, it seems plausible that in cases with subretinal hemorrhage involving the fovea, combined intravitreal administration of an anti-VEGF agent and expansile gas in order to attempt a rapid displacement of blood may have a beneficial effect.

Methods and Procedure

The procedure is performed under topical anesthesia with 2% lidocaine after preoperative antiseptic preparation which may be followed by neomycin sulfate drops. For anti-VEGF monotherapy, ranibizumab 0.5 mg or aflibercept 2 mg or bevacizumab 1.25 mg is injected intravitreally via the pars plana. Alternatively, anti-VEGF monotherapy may be combined with the intravitreal injection of expansile gas. After an aqueous tap to reduce intraocular pressure, 0.3–0.5 ml of 100% sulfur hexafluoride gas are injected into the vitreous cavity, followed by the injection of an anti-VEGF agent. Both injections are administered via the pars plana in the superotemporal or superonasal quadrant, 3–3.5 mm posterior to the limbus. Patients who received an additional hexafluoride gas injection are instructed to maintain prone positioning for 72 h. Repeated prone positioning may be extended for 24–48 h whenever blood displacement from under the fovea is not complete,.

Outcome

Several studies suggest that anti-VEGF monotherapy is a reasonable treatment option in patient's wet age-related macular degeneration associated with small subretinal macular hemorrhage [36–38]. The large-scale "Comparison of Age-Related Macular Degeneration Treatments Trials" (CATT) also included patients with subretinal hemorrhage who received anti-VEGF treatment. Results of this trial indicate that the eyes with neovascular AMD lesions composed of >50% blood can be managed similarly to those with less or no blood [36]. However, the major limitation of this study is hemorrhage size. The exclusion of patients with vitreous hemorrhage and patients with VA worse than 20/320 limits the generalizability of the CATT study findings. Because the great majority of patients (>92%) included in the CATT had hemorrhage sizes of ≤2 DA, this study hardly provides any information with regard to AMD in patients with large subretinal hemorrhages [38]. Unfortunately, this is exactly the subgroup of AMD patients with a poor prognosis and a high likelihood of identifying underlying risk factors for subretinal hemorrhage such as anticoagulant treatment or arterial hypertension.

The findings provided by the CATT are supported by our own observation in patients with small submacular hemorrhage secondary to exudative AMD who received anti-VEGF monotherapy (Figs. 5.5 and 5.6).

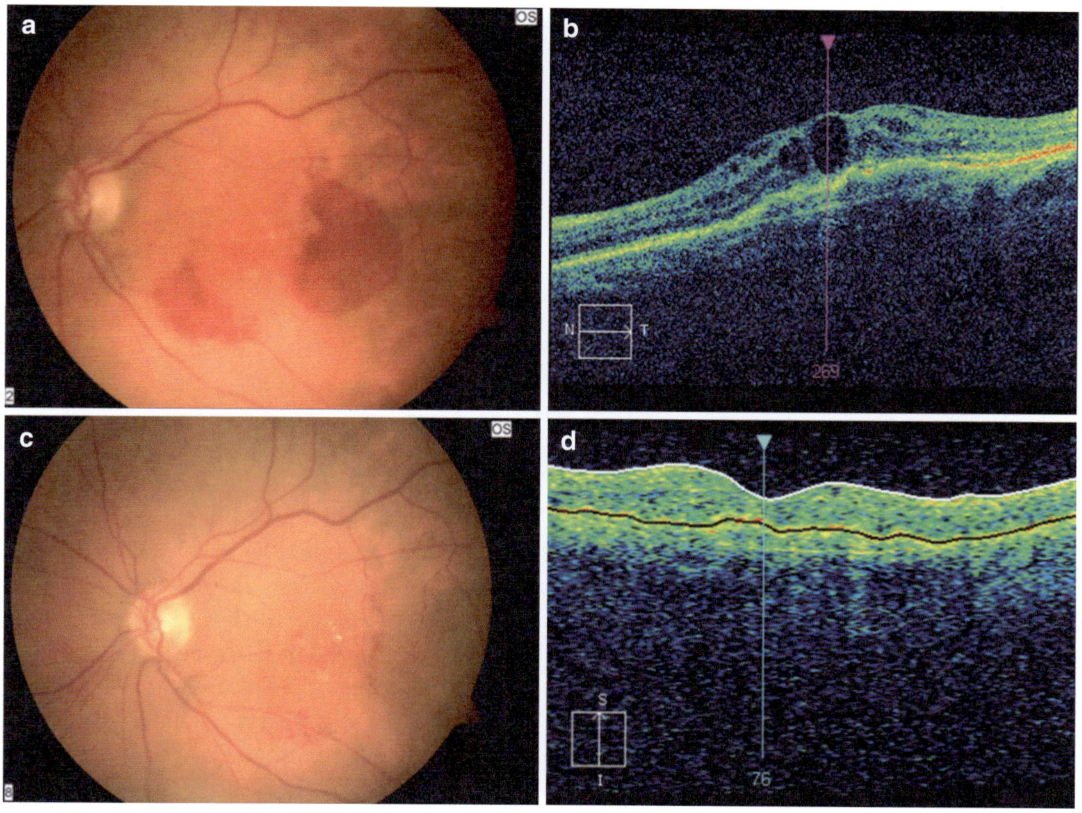

Fig. 5.5 (**a–d**) Fundus photographs and OCT of a patient with small subretinal hemorrhage (**a**, **b**), demonstrating almost complete resorption of blood and intraretinal fluid after three monthly injections of bevacizumab (**c**, **d**)

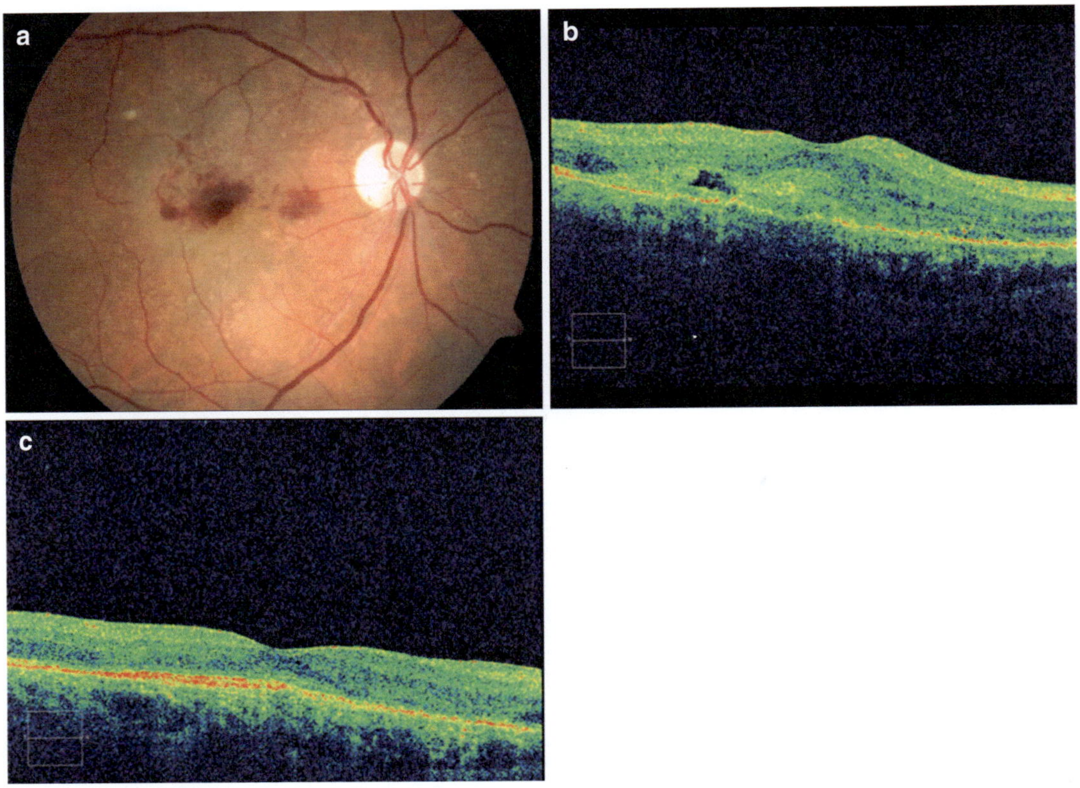

Fig. 5.6 (**a–c**) Fundus photograph and OCT of a patient with small (≤2 disc areas) subretinal hemorrhage (**a**, **b**). After three monthly injections of ranibizumab, we observed a complete resorption of blood and intraretinal fluid (**c**). Anti-VEGF monotherapy is a reasonable treatment option in patient's wet age-related macular degeneration associated with small subretinal macular hemorrhage

Other researchers compared the treatment outcomes of a combination of pneumatic displacement and intravitreal anti-VEGF and anti-VEGF monotherapy for submacular hemorrhage resulting from exudative age-related macular degeneration. In a retrospective case series, Shin and coworkers found that combination therapy showed a more rapid improvement of central foveal thickness within 1 month compared to monotherapy. Furthermore, visual outcome at 6 months was better in the combination therapy group in the eyes with subretinal hemorrhage thicker than 450 μm, whereas best-corrected visual acuity (BCVA) showed no significant difference between groups in the eyes with subretinal hemorrhage less than 450 μm. The authors concluded that both treatments are useful options for submacular hemorrhage resulting from exudative age-related macular degeneration, although combination therapy may yield a better treatment outcome than monotherapy in the eyes with thick subretinal hemorrhage [37].

The findings provided by Shin et al. are in accordance with our own results. In a recent study, we investigated the efficacy of combined intravitreal injection of bevacizumab and hexafluoride gas for submacular hemorrhage secondary to age-related macular degeneration [40]. In this case series, all patients received combined intravitreal injections with bevacizumab 1.25 mg and hexafluoride 0.3 mL. In each individual case, treatment with anti-VEGF drugs was continued as required. Time to treatment ranged from 1 to 4 weeks, and hemorrhage size ranged from 0.85 to 21.7 mm^2. Overall, displacement of blood was achieved in 80% of all cases. Visual acuity improved by three or more Snellen lines in 60%, remained stable in 30%, and worsened by three or more lines in 10%. Visual improvement compared to baseline was statistically significant. Following treatment with intravitreal bevacizumab and hexafluoride, 90% of all patients required additional injections with anti-VEGF agents, indicating that continued treatment of the underlying disorder is mandatory.

Combined Intravitreal Administration of rt-PA, Expansile Gas, and Anti-VEGF Agents with or Without Core Vitrectomy

With the advent of anti-VEGF agents and a rapid development of small-gauge transconjunctival vitreoretinal surgery, more complex minimally invasive approaches to the treatment of subretinal hemorrhage have become feasible.

Over the past years, several studies have demonstrated that 25 or 27 ga core vitrectomies, combined with pneumatic displacement with hexafluoride gas and intravitreal administration of rt-PA and anti-VEGF agents, have the potential to successfully treat even large subretinal hemorrhages, thereby avoiding the need for extensive vitreoretinal surgical procedures (Fig. 5.7). Interestingly, experimental studies have demonstrated that ranibizumab and bevacizumab can be coapplied with rt-PA as a treatment for neovascular age-related macular degeneration with submacular hemorrhage. Both ranibizumab and bevacizumab are not cleaved or functionally compromised by rt-PA or plasmin, whereas aflibercept is cleaved and its VEGF-binding ability is reduced when coapplied with plasmin [41, 42].

Methods and Procedure

The procedure is performed under topical and subconjunctival anesthesia with 2% lidocaine. Prior to injection, betadine is applied to the lids

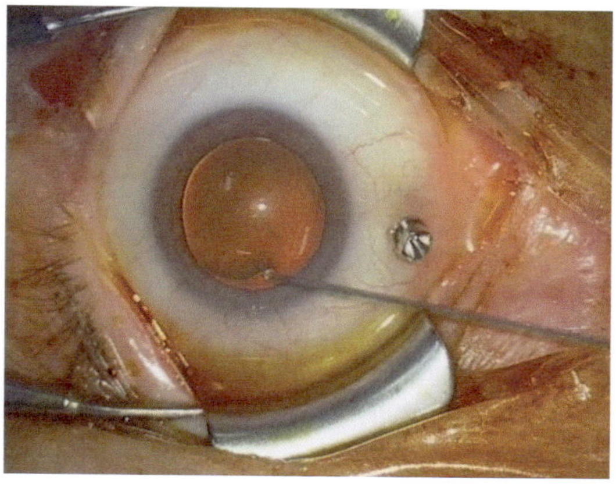

Fig. 5.7 27 Ga core vitrectomy and combined intravitreal administration of recombinant tissue-plasminogen activator (rt-PA), bevacizumab, and hexafluoride gas in a patient with subretinal hemorrhage secondary to wet age-related macular degeneration. Small-gauge sutureless transconjunctival core vitrectomy may be performed in combination with intravitreally injected drugs. To avoid reflux of injected drugs, the administration of rt-PA and bevacizumab should be performed after the injection of hexafluoride. Core vitrectomy has a beneficial effect on vitreous oxygenation and provides a reliable way to prevent increased postoperative intraocular pressure

and periorbita, and the eye is irrigated with sterile saline. A small-gauge (25 or 27 ga) trocar is then introduced through a beveled scleral incision 3.5 mm temporal to the limbus. After this, a core vitrectomy using a high-speed cutter (5000 cpm) is performed (Fig. 5.7). Then, 0.3–0.5 ml of 100% sulfur hexafluoride gas is injected through the pars plana port into the vitreous cavity.

Fifty micrograms of commercial rt-PA solution (Actilyse, Boehringer, Ingelheim, Germany) in a volume of 50 μL is drawn in a tuberculin syringe and injected into the midvitreous cavity through a 30-gauge needle, followed by the injection of an anti-VEGF agent, i.e., bevacizumab 1.25 mg or ranibizumab 0.5 mg. In order to avoid reflux of injected drugs, hexafluoride gas injection should be performed prior to the administration of rt-PA or anti-VEGF agents. To avoid hypotony, additional balanced saline solution (BSS) or hexafluoride gas may be injected into the vitreous cavity prior to removal of the pars plana port. Patients are then instructed to maintain prone positioning for 72 h. Whenever blood displacement from under the fovea is not complete, prone positioning may be extended for additional 24–48 h.

Outcome

Numerous studies have attempted to investigate the efficacy of combined treatment strategies in patients with macular hemorrhage using intravitreal rt-PA, expansile gas, and anti-VEGF agents with or without core vitrectomy. In a retrospective case series, Meyer et al. investigated the efficacy of combined intravitreal injection of rt-PA, bevacizumab, and hexafluoride gas in patients with subretinal hemorrhage secondary to AMD. After 3 months, they observed an average improvement in visual acuity from 20/133 to 20/74. None of their patients had reading vision prior to treatment, whereas 25% of all patients achieved reading vision at 1 month after treatment [43].

Thus far, several investigators reported on the use of small-gauge sutureless transconjunctival core vitrectomy which may be performed in combination with intravitreally injected drugs. Core vitrectomy has a beneficial effect on vitreous oxygenation and provides a reliable way to prevent increased postoperative intraocular pressure.

In a recent case series, Kadonosono and coworkers reported on a surgical procedure consisting of 25-gauge vitrectomy and submacular injection of 25 μg of rt-PA and 0.4 mL of air with a microneedle, followed by prone positioning overnight. Total subfoveal blood displacement was achieved in all 13 eyes and central lesion thickness decreased from a mean baseline value of 867 μm to a mean value of 379 μm at 1 month after surgery. Visual improvement was observed in 11 eyes, with a mean change in Early Treatment Diabetic Retinopathy Study letter score from baseline of 23.3 letters at 3 months. In one patient, however, postoperative formation of a macular hole was observed [44].

In another study, Ritzau-Tondrow et al. performed combined core vitrectomy and hexafluoride gas tamponade with subretinal injection of rt-PA and bevacizumab using a single pars plana incision. After an average follow-up period of 4.5 months, the authors observed an increase in visual acuity in 16 of 33 patients. Continued treatment with intravitreal anti-VEGF drugs was required in 14 cases. However, the authors also reported on two cases of postoperative retinal detachment that required buckling surgery [45].

From available studies, a minimally invasive approach based on intravitreal drug delivery appears to carry a lower risk of intra- or postoperative complications. To date, there is much evidence that intravitreal treatment of subretinal hemorrhage with recombinant tissue plasminogen activator (rt-PA), bevacizumab, and hexafluoride gas does not necessarily require the subretinal administration of drugs. In experimental studies, subretinal blood clots disappeared within 24 h after intravitreal administration of rt-PA, whereas there was no change in control eyes injected with saline solution [21]. Moreover, it has been demonstrated that albumin, a protein with a molecular weight similar to that of t-PA, is detectable in the subretinal space within 1 h, suggesting that rt-PA can migrate across the retina, thereby facilitating the dissolution of subretinal blood clots [22].

In a recent study, we investigated the efficacy of 27 or 25 ga core vitrectomy and combined intravitreal administration of recombinant tissue plasminogen activator (rt-PA), bevacizumab, and hexafluoride gas in patients with subretinal hemorrhage secondary to exudative age-related macular degeneration. This approach combines the beneficial effects of core vitrectomy, pneumatic displacement of subretinal blood, and simultaneous anti-VEGF treatment without touching the retina.

Patients treated in this series included cases with massive submacular hemorrhage secondary

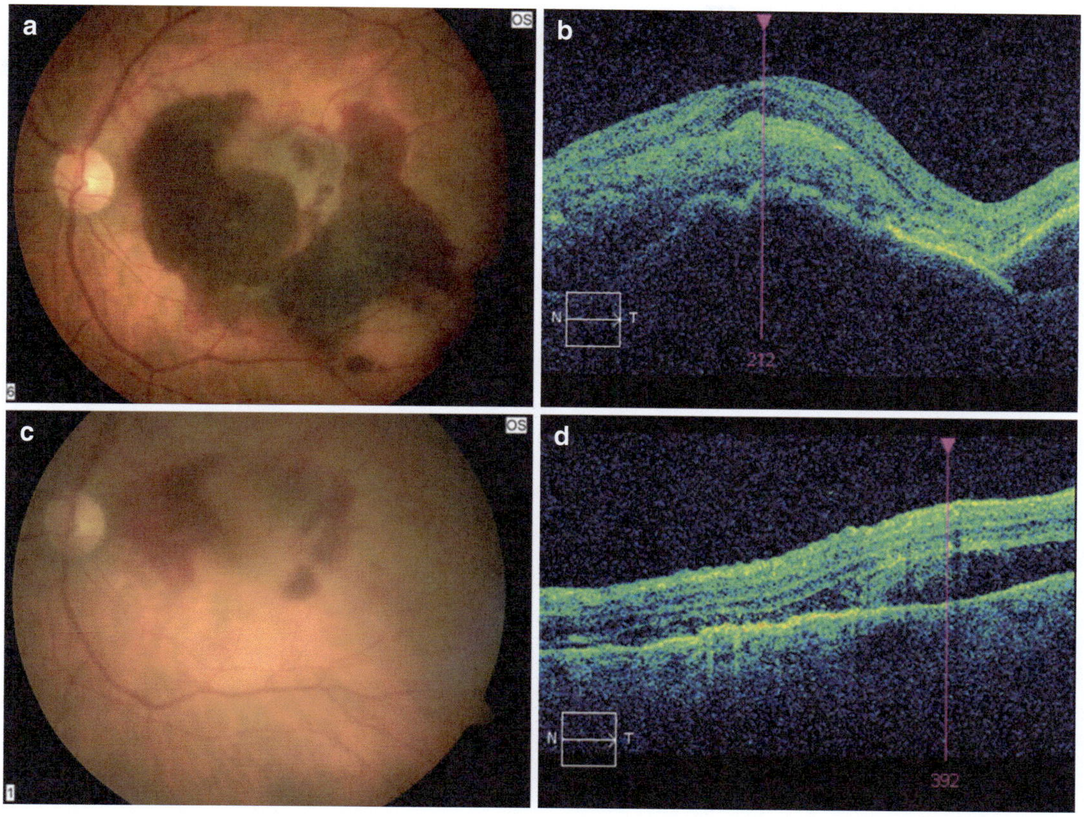

Fig. 5.8 (**a**, **b**) Preoperative fundus photograph and OCT of a 77-year-old patient with massive submacular hemorrhage secondary to age-related macular degeneration involving the fovea. (**c**, **d**) Fundus photograph and OCT 3 days after treatment with combined core vitrectomy and intravitreal rt-PA, bevacizumab, and hexafluoride gas, demonstrating a complete displacement from the center of the fovea and a significant reduction of central retinal thickness (CRT)

to age-related macular degeneration involving the fovea. We were able to demonstrate that core vitrectomy and combined intravitreal rt-PA, bevacizumab, and hexafluoride gas, followed by continued treatment with monthly intravitreal injections of bevacizumab, has the potential to result in complete displacement of massive subretinal hemorrhages from the center of the fovea, significant resorption of subretinal blood with reduction of central retinal thickness and visual improvement (Figs. 5.8 and 5.9). The proportion of patients with postoperative visual improvement of two or more Snellen lines was 52% and remained stable after continued treatment with intravitreal bevacizumab in 55.5% of all cases (Fig. 5.10). Complete displacement of blood from under the fovea was observed in 80% (Fig. 5.11).

These findings are not different in outcome compared to the results from other investigators who attempted a more invasive approach. In a retrospective study, Hillenkamp et al. investigated outcomes after vitrectomy, subretinal coapplication of rt-PA and bevacizumab, and hexafluoride gas tamponade, followed by postoperative PRN treatment with bevacizumab in 41 patients with submacular hemorrhage secondary to AMD. They observed a displacement of blood in 85%, and 29% of their patients achieved reading vision [46].

Chang and coworkers compared a combined treatment with vitrectomy, subretinal injection

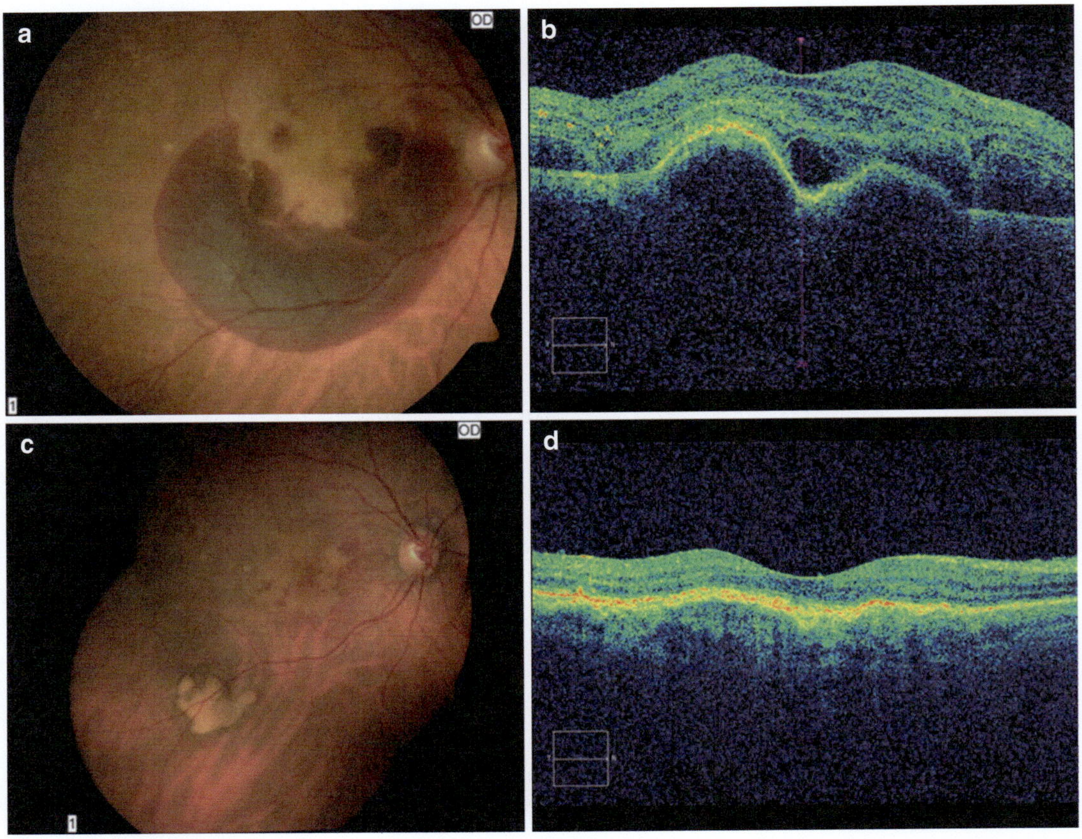

Fig. 5.9 (**a**, **b**) Preoperative fundus photograph and OCT of an 89-year-old patient with subretinal hemorrhage secondary to age-related macular degeneration and visual loss to 20/200. (**c**, **d**) Fundus photograph and OCT of the same eye 4 months after core vitrectomy, combined intravitreal injection of rt-PA, bevacizumab, and hexafluoride gas and continued treatment with monthly intravitreal injections of bevacizumab, demonstrating significant resorption of subretinal blood and complete displacement inferotemporal to the macula. By this time, visual acuity had improved to 20/60

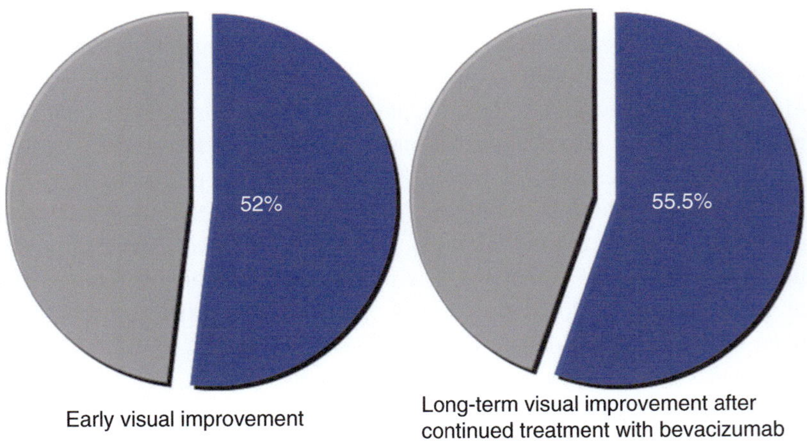

Fig. 5.10 Proportion of patients with postoperative visual improvement after core vitrectomy and combined intravitreal rt-PA, bevacizumab, and hexafluoride gas. Visual acuity improved two or more Snellen lines in 52% and remained stable after continued treatment with intravitreal bevacizumab in 55.5% of all cases

of rt-PA, and pneumatic displacement with or without postoperative anti-VEGF therapy. In their study, displacement of blood from under the fovea was observed in 81% and visual improvement of three or more Snellen lines in 19.6% of cases. After 6 months, the eyes that received postoperative anti-VEGF treatment exhibited better visual improvement compared to the group of eyes that did not receive postoperative anti-VEGF. Postoperative complications included vitreous hemorrhage in two eyes, rhegmatogenous retinal detachment in four eyes, and recurrent thick subretinal hemorrhage in six eyes [47].

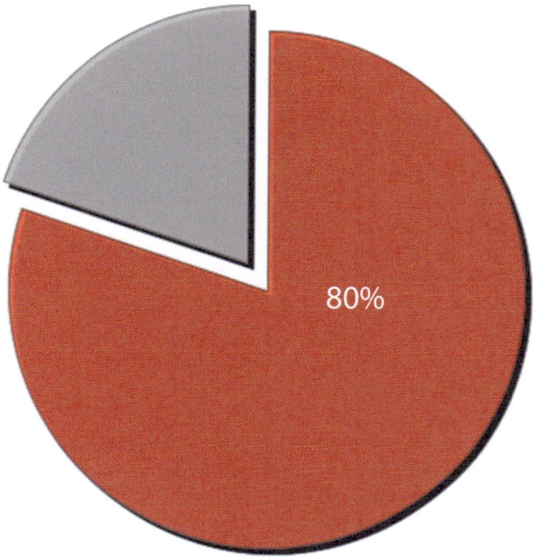

Fig. 5.11 After core vitrectomy and combined intravitreal rt-PA, bevacizumab, and hexafluoride gas, we observed a complete displacement of blood from under the fovea in 80% of cases

In the vast majority of cases, subretinal hemorrhage is associated with choroidal neovascularization secondary to exudative age-related macular degeneration. However, core vitrectomy and combined intravitreal rt-PA, bevacizumab, and hexafluoride gas also have been demonstrated to be a minimally invasive alternative to observation or surgical drainage or vitrectomy and subretinal injection of rt-PA in subretinal hemorrhage secondary to underlying conditions other than AMD [48]. Early pneumatic displacement is a useful treatment strategy in patients with thick contiguous subretinal or subhyaloidal blood that obscures the boundaries of a macroaneurysm amenable to further treatment with thermal photocoagulation (Fig. 5.12).

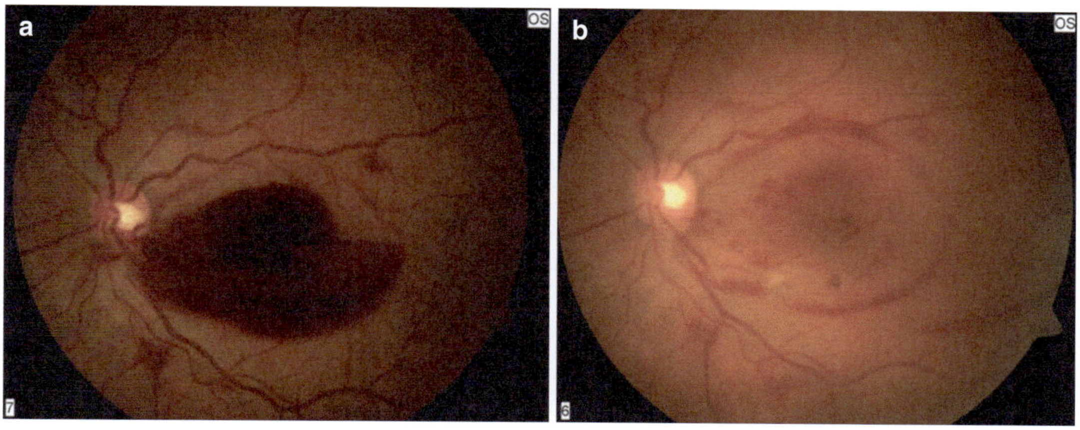

Fig. 5.12 (**a**) Fundus photograph of a 57-year-old female patient with acute visual loss (20/400) secondary to submacular-subhyaloidal hemorrhage of acute onset. (**b**) Fundus photograph after treatment with core vitrectomy and combined intravitreal rt-PA, bevacizumab, and hexafluoride gas and status post thermal photocoagulation of a retinal macroaneurysm. Visual acuity improved to 20/80. Early core vitrectomy with pneumatic displacement is a useful treatment strategy in patients with thick contiguous subretinal or subhyaloidal blood that obscures the boundaries of a macroaneurysm amenable to further treatment

References

1. Avery RL, Fekrat S, Hawkins BS, Bressler NM. Natural history of subfoveal subretinal hemorrhage in age-related macular degeneration. Retina. 1996;16:183–9.
2. Bennett SR, Folk JC, Blodi CF, Klugman M. Factors prognostic of visual outcome in patients with subretinal hemorrhage. Am J Ophthalmol. 1990;109:33–7.
3. Berrocal MH, Lewis ML, Flynn HW Jr. Variations in the clinical course of submacular hemorrhage. Am J Ophthalmol. 1996;122:486–93.
4. Wood WJ, Smith TR. Senile disciform macular degeneration complicated by massive hemorrhagic retinal detachment and angle closure glaucoma. Retina. 1983;3:296–303.
5. Scupola A, Coscas G, Soubrane G, Balestrazzi E. Natural history of macular subretinal hemorrhage in age-related macular degeneration. Ophthalmologica. 1999;213:97–102.
6. Glatt H, Machemer R. Experimental subretinal hemorrhage in rabbits. Ophthalmology. 1982;94:762–73.
7. Toth CA, Morse LS, Hjelmeland LM, Landers MB III. Fibrin directs early retinal damage after experimental subretinal hemorrhage. Arch Ophthalmol. 1991;109:723–9.
8. de Juan E Jr, Machemer R. Vitreous surgery for hemorrhagic and fibrous complications of age-related macular degeneration. Am J Ophthalmol. 1988;105:25–9.
9. Ibanez HE, Williams DF, Thomas MA, et al. Surgical management of submacular hemorrhage. Arch Ophthalmol. 1995;113:62–9.
10. Lim JI, Drews-Botsch C, Sternberg P Jr, et al. Submacular hemorrhage removal. Ophthalmology. 1995;102:1393–9.
11. Vander JF, Federman JL, Greven C, et al. Surgical removal of massive subretinal hemorrhage associated with age-related macular degeneration. Ophthalmology. 1991;98:23–7.
12. Kamei M, Tano Y, Maeno T, et al. Surgical removal of submacular hemorrhage using tissue plasminogen activator and perfluorocarbon liquid. Am J Ophthalmol. 1996;121:267–75.
13. Lewis H. Intraoperative fibrinolysis of submacular hemorrhage with tissue plasminogen activator and surgical drainage. Am J Ophthalmol. 1994;118:559–68.
14. Heriot WJ. Intravitreal gas and tPA: an outpatient procedure for submacular hemorrhage. Vail vitrectomy meeting, Vail, Colorado, 10–15 March 1996.
15. Benner JD, Hay A, Landers MB III, et al. Fibrinolytic-assisted removal of experimental subretinal hemorrhage within seven days reduces outer retinal degeneration. Ophthalmology. 1994;101:672–81.
16. Boone DE, Boldt HC, Ross RD, et al. The use of intravitreal tissue plasminogen activator in the treatment of experimental subretinal hemorrhage in the pig model. Retina. 1996;16:518–24.
17. Chaudhry NA, Mieler WF, Han DP, et al. Preoperative use of tissue plasminogen activator for large submacular hemorrhage. Ophthalmic Surg Lasers. 1999;30:176–80.
18. Jaffe GJ, Abrams GW, Williams GA, Han DP. Tissue plasminogen activator for postvitrectomy fibrin formation. Ophthalmology. 1990;97:184–9.
19. Jaffe GJ, Green GDJ, McKay BS, et al. Intravitreal clearance of tissue plasminogen activator in the rabbit. Arch Ophthalmol. 1988;106:969–72.
20. Morse LS, Benner JD, Hjelmeland LM, Landers MB III. Fibrinolysis of experimental subretinal haemorrhage without removal using tissue plasminogen activator. Br J Ophthalmol. 1996;80:658–62.
21. Coll GE, Sparrow JR, Marinovic A, Chang S. Effect of intravitreal tissue plasminogen activator on experimental subretinal hemorrhage. Retina. 1995;15:319–26.
22. Takeuchi A, Kricorian G, Yao XY, et al. The rate and source of albumin entry into saline-filled experimental retinal detachments. Invest Ophthalmol Vis Sci. 1994;35:3792–8.
23. Hesse L, Schroeder B, Heller G, Kroll P. Quantitative effect of intravitreally injected tissue plasminogen activator and gas on subretinal hemorrhage. Retina. 2000;20(5):500.
24. Hattenbach LO, Klais C, Koch FHJ, Gümbel HOC. Intravitreous injection of tissue plasminogen activator and gas in the treatment of submacular hemorrhage under various conditions. Ophthalmology. 2001;108:1485–92.
25. Hassan AS, Johnson MW, Schneiderman TE, et al. Management of submacular hemorrhage with intravitreous tissue plasminogen activator injection and pneumatic displacement. Ophthalmology. 1999;106:1900–6.
26. Hesse L, Schmidt J, Kroll P. Management of acute submacular hemorrhage using recombinant tissue plasminogen activator and gas. Graefes Arch Clin Exp Ophthalmol. 1999;237:273–7.
27. Johnson MW, Olsen KR, Hernandez E. Tissue plasminogen activator treatment of experimental subretinal hemorrhage. Retina. 1991;11:250–8.
28. Hrach CJ, Johnson MW, Hassan AS, et al. Retinal toxicity of commercial intravitreal tissue plasminogen activator solution in cat eyes. Arch Ophthalmol. 2000;118:659–63.
29. Ohji M, Saito Y, Hayashi A, et al. Pneumatic displacement of subretinal hemorrhage without tissue plasminogen activator. Arch Ophthalmol. 1998;116:1326–32.
30. Hattenbach LO, Brieden M, Koch F, Gümbel H. [Intravitreal injection of rt-PA and gas in the management of minor submacular haemorrhages secondary to age-related macular degeneration]. Klin Monbl Augenheilkd. 2002;219:512–8.
31. Lewis H, Resnick SC, Flannery JG, Straatsma BR. Tissue plasminogen activator treatment of experimental subretinal hemorrhage. Am J Ophthalmol. 1991;111:197–204.
32. Boyer DS, Antoszyk AN, Awh CC, Bhisitkul RB, Shapiro H, Acharya NR, MARINA Study Group. Subgroup analysis of the MARINA study of ranibizumab in neovascular age-related macular degeneration. Ophthalmology. 2007;114(2):246–52.

33. Brown DM, Michels M, Kaiser PK, Heier JS, Sy JP, Ianchulev T, ANCHOR Study Group. Ranibizumab versus verteporfin photodynamic therapy for neovascular age-related macular degeneration: two-year results of the ANCHOR study. Ophthalmology. 2009;116(1):57–65.
34. Rosenfeld PJ, Brown DM, Heier JS, Boyer DS, Kaiser PK, Chung CY, Kim RY, MARINA Study Group. Ranibizumab for neovascular age-related macular degeneration. N Engl J Med. 2006;355(14):1419–31.
35. Wolf S, Holz FG, Korobelnik JF, Lanzetta P, Mitchell P, Prünte C, Schmidt-Erfurth U, Weichselberger A, Hashad Y. Outcomes following three-line vision loss during treatment of neovascular age-related macular degeneration: subgroup analyses from MARINA and ANCHOR. Br J Ophthalmol. 2011;95(12):1713–8.
36. Altaweel MM, Daniel E, Martin DF, Mittra RA, Grunwald JE, Lai MM, Melamud A, Morse LS, Huang J, Ferris FL III, Fine SL, Maguire MG, Comparison of Age-related Macular Degeneration Treatments Trials (CATT) Research Group; Comparison of Age-related Macular Degeneration Treatments Trials CATT Research Group. Outcomes of eyes with lesions composed of >50% blood in the Comparison of Age-related Macular Degeneration Treatments Trials (CATT). Ophthalmology. 2015;122(2):391–8.
37. Shin JY, Lee JM, Byeon SH. Anti-vascular endothelial growth factor with or without pneumatic displacement for submacular hemorrhage. Am J Ophthalmol. 2015;159(5):904–14.
38. Ying GS, Maguire MG, Daniel E, Grunwald JE, Ahmed O, Martin DF. Comparison of Age-Related Macular Degeneration Treatments Trials Research Group. Association between antiplatelet or anticoagulant drugs and retinal or subretinal hemorrhage in the Comparison of Age-Related Macular Degeneration Treatments Trials. Ophthalmology. 2016;123(2):352–60.
39. Sharei V, Höhn F, Köhler T, Hattenbach LO, Mirshahi A. Course of intraocular pressure after intravitreal injection of 0.05 mL ranibizumab (Lucentis). Eur J Ophthalmol. 2010;20(1):174–9.
40. Höhn F, Mirshahi A, Hattenbach LO. [Combined intravitreal injection of bevacizumab and SF6 gas for treatment of submacular hemorrhage secondary to age-related macular degeneration]. Ophthalmologe. 2010;107(4):328–32.
41. Klettner A, Grotelüschen S, Treumer F, Roider J, Hillenkamp J. Compatibility of recombinant tissue plasminogen activator (rtPA) and aflibercept or ranibizumab coapplied for neovascular age-related macular degeneration with submacular haemorrhage. Br J Ophthalmol. 2015;99(6):864–9.
42. Klettner A, Puls S, Treumer F, Roider J, Hillenkamp J. Compatibility of recombinant tissue plasminogen activator and bevacizumab co-applied for neovascular age-related macular degeneration with submacular hemorrhage. Arch Ophthalmol. 2012;130(7):875–81.
43. Meyer CH, Scholl HP, Eter N, Helb HM, Holz FG. Combined treatment of acute subretinal haemorrhages with intravitreal recombined tissue plasminogen activator, expansile gas and bevacizumab: a retrospective pilot study. Acta Ophthalmol. 2008; 86(5):490–4.
44. Kadonosono K, Arakawa A, Yamane S, Inoue M, Yamakawa T, Uchio E, Yanagi Y. Displacement of submacular hemorrhages in age-related macular degeneration with subretinal tissue plasminogen activator and air. Ophthalmology. 2015;122(1):123–8.
45. Ritzau-Tondrow U, Baraki H, Hoerauf H. [Minimally invasive therapy of submacular hemorrhage in exsudative age-related macular degeneration]. Ophthalmologe. 2012;109(7):670–5.
46. Hillenkamp J, Klettner A, Puls S, Treumer F, Subretinal RJ. co-application of rtPA and bevacizumab for exudative AMD with submacular hemorrhage. Compatibility and clinical long-term results. Ophthalmologe. 2012;109(7):648–56.
47. Chang W, Garg SJ, Maturi R, Hsu J, Sivalingam A, Gupta SA, Regillo CD, Ho AC. Management of thick submacular hemorrhage with subretinal tissue plasminogen activator and pneumatic displacement for age-related macular degeneration. Am J Ophthalmol. 2014;157(6):1250–7.
48. Hillenkamp J, Surguch V, Framme C, Gabel VP, Sachs HG. Management of submacular hemorrhage with intravitreal versus subretinal injection of recombinant tissue plasminogen activator. Graefes Arch Clin Exp Ophthalmol. 2010;248(1):5–11.

Surgical and Nonsurgical Treatment of Pre-retinal Hemorrhages

6

Gerald Seidel and Anton Haas

Introduction

A pre-retinal hemorrhage is the accumulation of blood between the internal limiting membrane (ILM) and the posterior vitreous hyaloid. Some authors incorrectly expand the term to hemorrhages underneath the ILM, where it constitutes a misnomer; these hemorrhages are truly intraretinal because the ILM is part of the retina. Nevertheless this chapter will discuss both true pre-retinal and sub-ILM hemorrhages, since the two cannot always be discriminated with certainty and many treatment concepts are, with minor adaptions, equally applicable to both of them.

Pre-retinal and sub-ILM hemorrhages lead to a sudden loss of vision where the retina is blocked and are as such severely debilitating, especially when they are located in front of the macula. However, some patients experience also more peripheral hemorrhages as a heavy burden, particularly those with long-standing macular pathologies like an ischemic diabetic maculopathy. Figure 6.1 shows an acute case of a pre-retinal hemorrhage covering the macula.

There is a plethora of causes of pre-retinal and sub-ILM hemorrhages including valsalva retinopathy, Terson's syndrome, macroaneurysms, blunt trauma, traumatic laser injury, hematologic disorders, and proliferative retinopathies as seen in diabetes, retinal vein and artery occlusions, retinopathy of prematurity, and vasculitis [1–8]. While some pathologies tend to cause rather one or the other location of hemorrhage, some can cause both. For example, hemorrhages due to proliferative retinopathies tend to be truly pre-retinal, while hemorrhages in Terson's syndrome or macroaneurysms frequently also induce sub-ILM hemorrhages. In children the hemorrhages under the ILM predominate because of this population's strong adhesion of the vitreoretinal interface. This either confines the hemorrhage underneath the ILM or leads the blood to break into the vitreous without detaching the posterior hyaloid [9–12]. Similarly, hemorrhages in valsalva retinopathy also tend to accumulate under the ILM rather than under the posterior hyaloid, but the data on this pathology are particularly scarce [13–16].

The paucity of data is a general issue of pre-retinal hemorrhages and makes the choice of the optimal treatment difficult. So far there are no published randomized clinical trials dealing with the treatment for pre-retinal hemorrhages. Thus it needs to be considered that most of the information that follows relies on often small, mostly retrospective case series without a control group. To add confusion, the term pre-retinal is sometimes arbitrarily applied to include not only sub-ILM and sub-hyaloidal hemorrhages but also

G. Seidel, M.D., P.D., Dr.Sc., F.E.B.O. (✉)
A. Haas, M.D., P.D.
Department of Ophthalmology, Medical University of Graz/Austria, Graz, Austria
e-mail: gerald.seidel@medunigraz.at

L.-O. Hattenbach (ed.), *Management of Macular Hemorrhage*,
https://doi.org/10.1007/978-3-319-65877-3_6

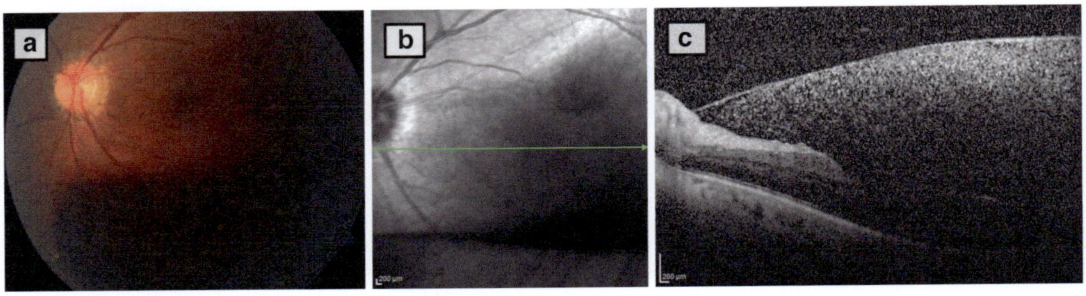

Fig. 6.1 Acute pre-retinal hemorrhage. A 3-day-old pre-retinal hemorrhage in a diabetic patient shows an incipient sedimentation of the blood at the inferior boarder of the pre-retinal space formed by the incomplete vitreous detachment on a color fundus image (**a**) and on an infrared image (**b**). Albeit a faint contour of the fovea can be made out on OCT (**c**) even such a relatively mild hemorrhage significantly obscures the retinal details

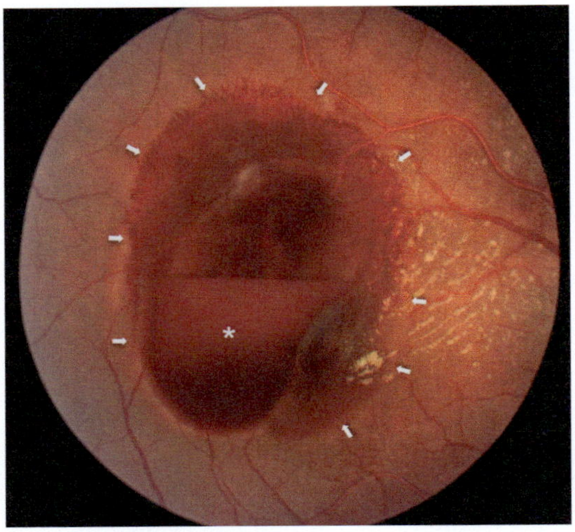

Fig. 6.2 Retinal macroaneurysm. The fundus image shows a classic presentation of a retinal macroaneurysm with the triad of a subretinal hemorrhage (arrows) encompassing almost the entire macular area, an intraretinal hemorrhage, and a pre-retinal hemorrhage (asterisk). The yellow deposits nasally are hard exudates

intravitreal hemorrhages. Most diseases leading to pre-retinal hemorrhages simultaneously cause other pathologies in the eye such as intravitreal and intraretinal hemorrhages, retinal ischemia, or vitreoretinal traction. For example, a macroaneurysm typically presents with a triad of subretinal, intraretinal, and pre-retinal hemorrhage (Fig. 6.2). A dense pre-retinal sheet of blood might obscure any retinal pathology that ultimately limits the visual outcome regardless of the treatment for the pre-retinal pathology. Thus, the potential influence of comorbidities on the outcome of any treatment should be considered when reviewing the literature and when choosing the treatment for an individual patient.

This chapter gives an overview about the current available options, their advantages, and drawbacks, and it also points out special considerations that might apply to specific diseases. It should serve as a guide to the practitioner for informing and treating patients in the light of the evidence available.

Observation

A treatment for a pre-retinal hemorrhage is not always necessary. This holds true for both sub-ILM and sub-hyaloidal hemorrhages [17].

For both types of hemorrhages the time to complete reabsorption is highly variable, and while some resolve within a few months, in others visually significant remnants of blood can persist for decades. In a retrospective case series on the natural history in Terson's syndrome, one sub-hyaloidal hemorrhage had resolved within 4 months and another still persisted after 13 years of follow-up [17]. Another group reported an average time of 8.7 months to reach the best final visual acuity in untreated cases of Terson's syndrome with a dome-shaped pre-retinal hemorrhage, which presumably represented the cases with a sub-ILM and/or a sub-hyaloidal hemorrhage. In the same study, the patients with denser dome-shaped hemorrhages (70%) received a vitrectomy. It took these patients on average 9.4

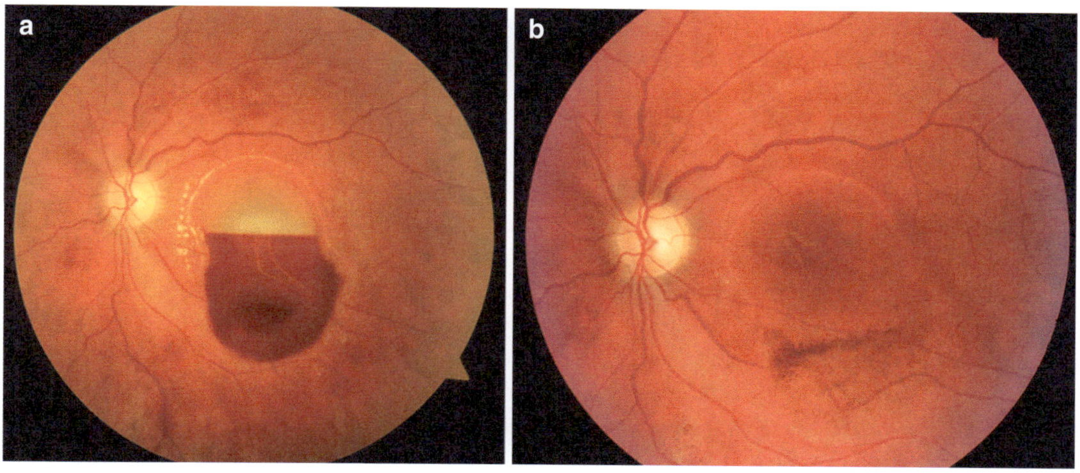

Fig. 6.3 Spontaneous resolution of a pre-retinal hemorrhage. A poorly controlled hypertonic patient reported a sudden drop of vision on the left eye 1 month ago. His visual acuity was reduced to 20/200 due to a dens already partially dehemoglobinized pre-retinal hemorrhage (**a**). After 3 months of observation the hemorrhage had almost completely resolved and vision had improved to 20/25 with some residual subfoveal RPE mottling (**b**)

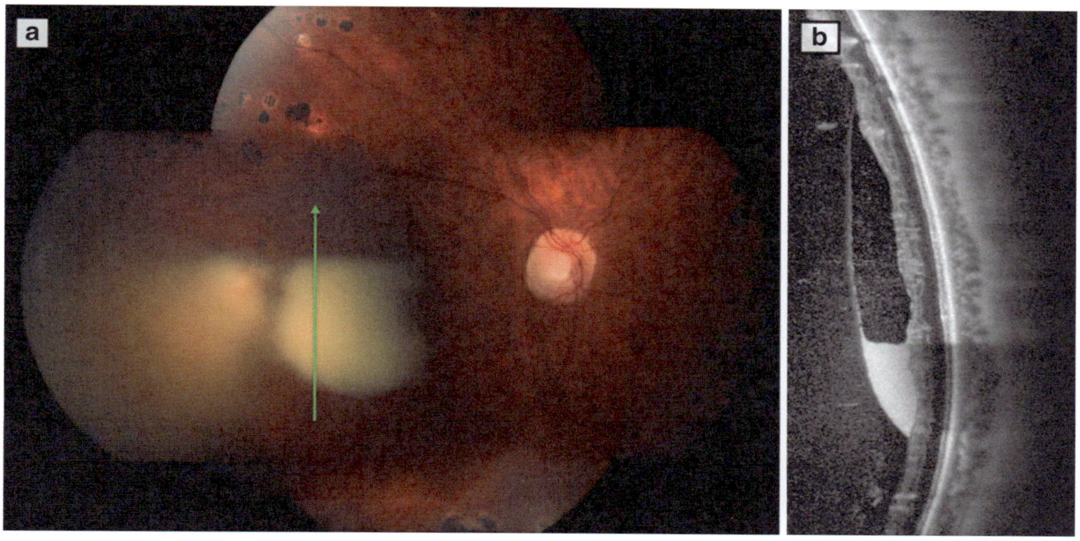

Fig. 6.4 Long-standing pre-retinal hemorrhage. (**a**) Shows a diabetic fundus with an untreated 2-year-old parafoveal pre-retinal hemorrhage, which due to its dehemoglobinized state has turned yellow. The patient did not feel bothered by the paracentral nasal scotoma and visual acuity remained around 20/25 throughout the observation period. An OCT of the same hemorrhage 1 year later (**b**) shows the partial reabsorption of the blood. Note the non-central retinal atrophy due to ischemia

months to recover their best visual acuity [18]. In a prospective case series on vitreous hemorrhage in Terson's syndrome 60% resolved spontaneously within 3 months. How many of these cases included pre-retinal hemorrhages was not specified [19]. Similar to these data on Terson's syndrome, the data on the dynamics of spontaneous resolution of hemorrhages due to other pathologies vary from a few weeks to many years [20]. Figure 6.3 shows a case of almost complete spontaneous resolution of a pre-retinal hemorrhage in a hypertensive patient within 3 months. Figure 6.4 showcases an exceedingly slow and incomplete resolution over 3 years.

In cases of persisting blood, the accumulation of breakdown products close to the delicate tissue of the retina poses the question of potential toxic retinal damage. While the retinal toxicity of extravasal blood under and in the retina has been shown [21], it seems to be, if at all, much less of an issue for pre-retinal and sub-ILM hemorrhages. This is supported by normal values of retinal sensitivity measured by micro fundus perimetry after the resolution of sub-ILM hemorrhages in pathologies without an underlying retinal damage. These findings were independent from the size or the treatment of the hemorrhage [22]. Further, excellent visual outcomes for sub-ILM and sub-hyaloidal hemorrhages have been reported even when surgery was delayed for over 6 months or a spontaneous resolution had been awaited for years [17, 23].

In contrast to retinal toxicity, the concern for a higher risk of epiretinal membrane (ERM) growth seems to be more justified. In animal models an ERM formation can be consistently triggered by inducing a pre-retinal hemorrhage with a laser or by the repeated intravitreal injection of blood [24, 25]. However, for humans there still is controversy over the role of blood in the formation of ERMs, and the incidence of ERMs after pre-retinal hemorrhages varies significantly. Table 6.1 shows the incidence of ERM formation in Terson's syndrome and valsalva retinopathy for untreated and treated patients. It also highlights the heterogeneity of the data regarding their account on the hemorrhage localization and regarding the follow-up. ERMs are not unique to untreated cases. In a report from 1991, all patients with presumably either a sub-ILM or sub-hyaloidal hemorrhage (the authors used the term hemorrhagic macular cyst) developed an ERM within 2 years, regardless if they were observed or a vitrectomy had been performed. None of the treated eyes received any kind of membrane peeling at the time of the initial surgery. Albeit their incidence was high, most of these ERMs were visually insignificant [18]. Figure 6.5 shows an example of an ERM formation after a vitrectomy for a non-clearing severe pre-retinal hemorrhage.

Aside from the blood triggering a formation of ERMs, there are other potential factors such as damage from acutely elevated intraocular pressure in Terson's syndrome and valsalva retinopathy. In diabetics and in patients with retinal vein occlusions, the formation of secondary ERMs even in the absence of a pre-retinal hemorrhage is

Table 6.1 The incidence of epiretinal membranes after sub-hyaloidal and sub-inner limiting membrane hemorrhage

Trial	Disease	Incidence of ERM % (no. of events/total no. of patients)		Mean follow-up (months)	Comments
		Observation	Intervention		
Schulz et al. [18]	Terson's	100% (3/3)	100% (7/7) PPV[a] 3 months after onset	50	Subgroup analysis of sub-hyaloidal hemorrhages
Kuhn et al. [10]	Terson's	18% (6/33)[b] Intra-OP[c] (mean after 6 months)	0% (0/13) PPV[a] + ERM/ILM peeling[d]	26	Subgroup analysis of "hemorrhagic macular cyst"
Skevas et al. [19]	Terson's	20% (4/20)[b] Intra-OP[c] (mean after 4.4 months)	0% (0/20)[b] PPV[a] + ERM/ILM peeling[d]	6.4 (postop)	Hemorrhage not specified
Stiebel-Kalish et al. [17]	Terson's	0% (0/12)	NA	57	Non traumatic sub-hyaloidal hemorrhages
Durukan et al. [37]	Valsalva retinopathy	NA	0% (0/16) Nd:YAG membranotomy	24	Sub-ILM; mean time to treatment less than 6 days

[a]Pars plana vitrectomy
[b]Type of hemorrhage (sub-ILM, sub-hyaloidal, intravitreal) not specified
[c]Intraoperative fundus assessment
[d]Epiretinal membrane and inner limiting membrane peeling

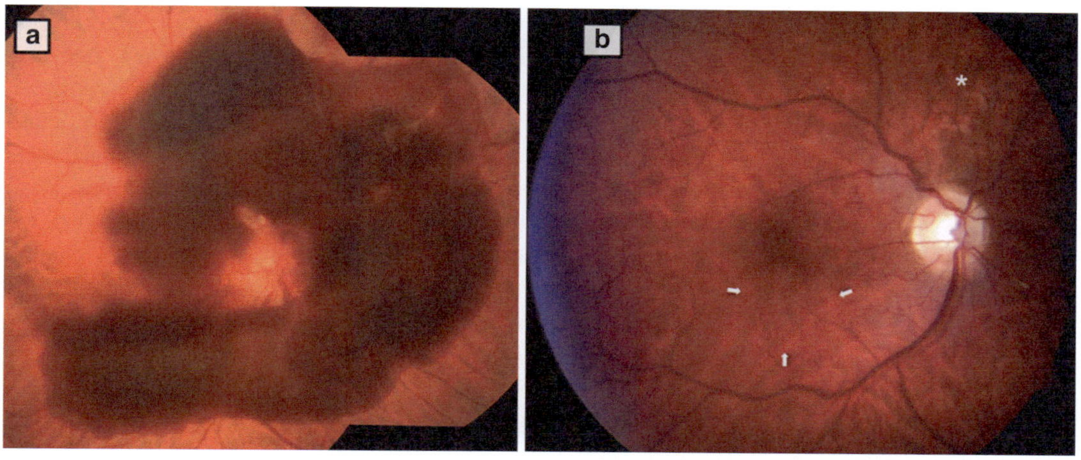

Fig. 6.5 Vitrectomy for a non-clearing pre-retinal hemorrhage: a 7-year follow-up. A 50-year-old hypertensive patient presented with a sudden spontaneous drop of vision to 20/200 with an extensive pre-retinal hemorrhage involving most of the posterior pole (**a**). After 1 week of observation, the blood dispersed into the vitreous, and the patient experienced an additional deterioration of his visual acuity to light perception. Since the vitreous hemorrhage subsequently failed to reabsorb, 6 months after the initial presentation, a vitrectomy was performed. Due to a postoperative retinal detachment, the procedure was revised with an encircling band, endolaser, and a C3F8 gas tamponade. The patient regained a visual acuity of 20/20. The fundus 7 years after the procedure (**b**) shows a delicate paracentral epiretinal membrane (ERM; arrows) and some mottling of the RPE superior to the optic disk (asterisk). Similar to most cases in the literature, aside from the pre-retinal hemorrhage, other factors could explain both the ERM and the RPE mottling

relatively common [26]. This complicates the risk analysis in these diseases.

Other than ERMs, pathologies associated less frequently with pre-retinal hemorrhages are pigmentary maculopathy and macular holes. Pigmentary changes at the level of retinal pigment epithelium have been reported in eyes with pre-retinal hemorrhages in Terson's syndrome both without treatment and after 12 month deferred vitrectomy [10, 17]. If these changes are truly caused by the pre-retinal hemorrhage, or if the pre-retinal hemorrhage solely obscured a deeper pathology is unclear.

Similarly, macular holes after pre-retinal hemorrhages could only be identified after the spontaneous resolution or the surgical removal of the blood. While some reports explicitly excluded traumatic causes of the hemorrhage [27], others did not [1], which leaves the possibility of a traumatic origin of the hole in the latter. The single reported macular hole after a sub-ILM hemorrhage in valsalva retinopathy had a peculiar configuration with an intact ILM preventing the hole from enlarging. The eye was left untreated and after 9 months had regained a visual acuity of 20/25, which subsequently remained stable for at least 8 months [28]. Taken together, macular holes are exceedingly rare complications of pre-retinal hemorrhages and depending on the anatomical configuration might be observed without immediate intervention.

Observation is less of an option in pediatric cases. If treatment is deferred, young children can rapidly develop amblyopia. Unfortunately, even after a prompt removal of the blood, the prognosis remains guarded. In children a sub-ILM or intravitreal hemorrhage often reflects a severe retinal disease or injury [29, 30]. In addition to the ocular damage, many pediatric cases of traumatic vitreous hemorrhage are associated with severe accidental and non-accidental head trauma. The resulting brain damage often plays a significant role in a persistent visual dysfunction [10, 31].

In general, if the underlying pathology warrants an early intervention or if visually significant remnants of the blood persist, treatment is indicated.

Laser

The perforation of the posterior hyaloid by a laser as treatment for pre-retinal hemorrhages was first reported in 1980 by Fechner et al., who used an argon laser for this purpose [32]. Some recent reports also advocate this approach with good results, but retinal scaring as a complication has been noted [33, 34]. Despite its long history and the rekindled interest in argon laser membranotomy, it has been rarely used after the report on Nd:YAG membranotomy by Faulborn in 1988 [35]. The latter provides a treatment option for both sub-ILM and sub-hyaloidal hemorrhages due to a variety of causes including diabetic retinopathy, valsalva retinopathy, Terson's syndrome, retinal vein occlusion, and hematologic disorders [3, 36–38]. The concept comprises giving the blood trapped underneath the ILM or posterior hyaloid a path to escape into the vitreous and thus freeing the fovea from the dense cover of blood. Thereby the visual recovery of the patient and the visualization of the retina are expedited. However, if the blood truly clears faster from the eye when it is diluted in the vitreous or if the reabsorption is actually impaired remains to be elucidated.

This procedure typically uses a Q-switched Nd:YAG laser in single burst mode. After the visualization of the fundus with, for example, a Goldmann three-mirror lens, single shots ranging around 2.5–10.0 mJ are applied. A good pupil dilation minimizes the energy needed, and often one to ten shots are sufficient to achieve a pertinent opening. Ideally the puncture should be placed neither directly over the fovea nor superiorly but rather at the inferior slant of the hemorrhagic dome to facilitate the gravitational drainage of the blood. Attention must be paid if there is a sufficiently thick blood column at the site of the treatment to shield the retina from the laser. An unshielded Nd:YAG laser aimed 2 mm in front of the retina with the energy typically needed for a successful membranotomy will consistently produce a retinal damage in monkeys and rabbits [39].

If performed correctly, complications after Nd:YAG membranotomy are rare. In one case of valsalva retinopathy, the induction of a macular hole has been reported for a foveal, one disk diameter, sub-ILM hemorrhage [36]. As previously discussed sub-ILM hemorrhages by definition block the view to the structures underneath and can themselves cause macular holes. So if this complication can be truly attributed to the treatment is uncertain. Nevertheless, caution when applying the laser should be exercised, and we recommend starting with low-energy settings and increasing the energy in small increments if needed. One should choose the location of treatment carefully; a thicker shield of blood might prevent retinal damage, and thus we preferentially use Nd:YAG membranotomy in larger hemorrhages, that is, larger than three disk diameters [36, 37].

Another potential complication is ERMs. Though their formation months after Nd:YAG membranotomy has been described in case reports [14], the incidence seems lower than when a spontaneous reabsorption is awaited. In a case series on 16 eyes with valsalva retinopathy, a Nd:YAG membranotomy was performed within 16 days from the symptom's onset. None of the eyes developed an epiretinal membrane within the 2-year follow-up [37]. Similar results were obtained in a smaller study on five eyes treated within 24 hours [16]. In some cases of sub-ILM hemorrhages the partially detached ILM fails to reattach to the retinal surface and can subsequently partially contract. This usually is visually insignificant [40].

While most eyes without a proliferative retinopathy tend to recover good visual acuity without the need for further interventions after the Nd:YAG membranotomy [36, 37], the data on patients with a proliferative retinopathy are mixed. A major issue is the reabsorption of the induced vitreous hemorrhage. Whereas one series reported resolution in all of its nine treated proliferative diabetic eyes [41], another series that included nine patients with proliferative retinopathy (5 diabetics and 5 branch retinal vein occlsions) reported that five (55%) of these eyes subsequently required a vitrectomy. After a successful membranotomy in all these cases, the blood failed to reabsorb in the vitreous, and, in addition to that, one patient developed a retinal detachment and another an ERM [36].

The following special considerations for Nd:YAG membranotomies in proliferative retinopathies are important. First, if needed a panretinal or sectorial laser should precede the membranotomy. The Nd:YAG laser effectively induces a vitreous hemorrhage that might prohibit prompt and efficient retinal photocoagulation. In the pre-anti-VEGF era deferral of the panretinal photocoagulation was sometimes advocated to treat a potential diabetic macular edema first [41], but this does not hold when intravitreal treatment is available. Second, one can assume intravitreal blood and its catabolic products induce changes in the vitreous gel. This has the potential for aggravating vitreoretinal tractions, which are the cause of the bleeding to begin with [42]. As such, severe proliferative vitreoretinopathy has been described in dens vitreous hemorrhages in a case series on non-traumatic Terson's syndrome [43]. The physician and the patient should be aware of this risk, and patients with severe tractions should be closely monitored if a Nd:YAG membranotomy is decided on.

A successful puncture of the posterior hyaloid and sometimes also ILM is usually apparent right after the laser shot, but sometimes the blood clings to the retinal surface despite multiple obviously pertinent membranotomies. This signals most probably that the blood has clotted. While laser treatment is frustrating in these cases, these clots tend to stick rather firmly to the posterior hyaloid and offer little resistance when being removed while inducing a posterior vitreous detachment during vitrectomy. It follows that Nd:YAG membranotomy should be performed before clotting has occurred. The window of opportunity is ill defined, but most laser-refractory cases were treated later than 1 month from symptom onset [36, 44].

In cases where a dispersion of blood into the vitreous was achieved, the visual recovery tends to be within days to 1 month [36, 38, 45]. The timeframe again is hard to predict and might depend on the vitreous configuration, with a detached or more liquefied vitreous leading to faster diffusion and thus faster recovery compared to eyes with an attached posterior hyaloid and a firmer vitreous gel [38]. Figure 6.6 demonstrates the resolution of a sub-ILM hemorrhage after an uncomplicated Nd:YAG membranotomy.

Despite good results in many instances, when Nd:YAG membranotomy does not sufficiently address the companioning pathologies, as well as when significant intraocular hemorrhage persists or recurs another treatment approach should step in.

Vitrectomy

In the 1980s, dense pre-macular hemorrhages used to make up around 6% of primary vitrectomy cases [46]. The relative incidence has certainly shifted since then due to a broadening of indications for vitrectomy, but some cases with pre-retinal hemorrhage, especially diabetics, still require surgery. Not only is a vitrectomy the most reliable way to remove the hemorrhage, but it also releases vitreoretinal tractions, which in proliferative cases play an important pathogenic role in the bleeding. A simultaneously applied epiretinal membrane and ILM peeling, panretinal photocoagulation, intravitreal drug delivery, and gas or oil tamponades can reduce the risk of long-term sequel such as epiretinal membrane formation or ERM recurrence, cystoid macular edema, new neovascularization, and recurrent hemorrhage.

The point of time for a vitrectomy needs to be individually chosen. Due to comorbidities some patients may present late, like those with Terson's syndrome, many of whom will not make it to an ophthalmologist at all because of severe neurologic sequela or death [47]. As such, intraocular hemorrhage is a known independent risk factor for a higher mortality and long-term morbidity in patients with non-traumatic subarachnoidal hemorrhages [48]. This is not to say that late-presenting patients lack the potential for significant visual improvement by a vitrectomy even after a long-standing pre-retinal deposition of blood. As noted earlier, there is hardly any evi-

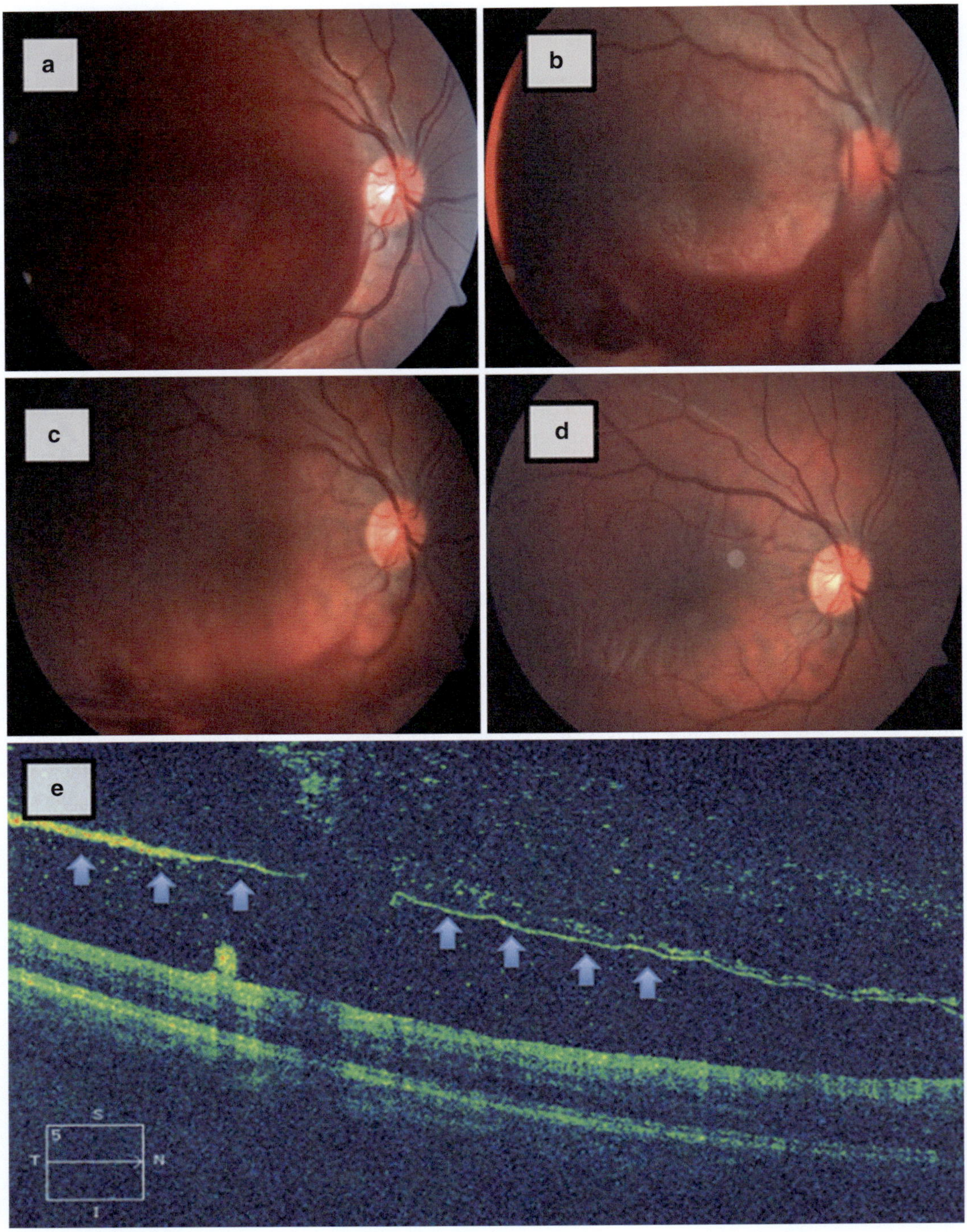

Fig. 6.6 Nd:YAG membranotomy for valsalva retinopathy. A previously healthy 22-year-old pregnant patient presented because of a drop in vision to counting fingers after repeated emesis 4 days prior. Fundus examination revealed a large presumably sub-ILM hemorrhage (**a**), which was treated after a thorough discussion of all therapeutic options by Nd:YAG membranotomy (three shots; 2,4 mJ maximal energy). Already 5 min after the treatment, most of the blood had dispersed into the vitreous (**b**) and vision increased to 20/40 after 3 days (**c**) and 20/20 after 1 month (**d**). The pertinent membranotomy in the still elevated partially thickened ILM (arrows) can be seen on SD-OCT taken 3 days after the laser (**e**)

dence for retinal toxicity in these cases, and excellent visual results have been achieved after a late vitrectomy.

Apart from the cases where an early intervention is not an option, the previously recommended waiting periods around 6–12 months in nonproliferative pre-retinal hemorrhages fail to reflect common practice today [49]; as the surgical techniques have become ever more refined, many surgeons are less hesitant to intervene. This is also true for the Diabetic Retinopathy Vitrectomy Study's recommendations on vitreous hemorrhage in proliferative diabetic retinopathy, which basically concluded that an early vitrectomy in type II diabetes did not translate into better visual outcomes than if the vitrectomy was deferred. However, type I diabetes profited significantly form an earlier intervention. The hypothesis for the discording results between the two groups was a presumably more active disease in type I diabetes [50]. Arguably, a pre-retinal hemorrhage is a sign of disease activity in proliferative diabetic retinopathy, and an earlier vitrectomy for these eyes regardless of the type of diabetes has been suggested [46, 51]. Yet, none of these latter studies were randomized clinical controlled trials, and we are currently lacking hard evidence regarding the optimal time to intervene for diabetic pre-retinal hemorrhages.

Above all, a vitrectomy carries certain risks for the patient. It might induce cataract progression, retinal breaks, or endophthalmitis; postoperative rebleeding occurs in 13–61% of diabetic vitrectomies [52–54]. The rates are similar when silicone oil is used, but the hemorrhages tend to stay confined to a smaller area, which might on the one hand be less debilitating for the patient but might on the other hand induce fibrotic pre-retinal proliferations which require additional surgery [55]. There is mounting evidence that the severity of intraoperative and postoperative bleeding can be reduced with the intravitreal injection of anti-VEGF agents prior to surgery [56].

Conversely, after a vitrectomy, the intravitreal application of medications might lose some of their effect. This is especially an issue of anti-VEGF agents where the intraocular half-life is reduced sevenfold [57]; it is a lesser problem of intravitreal steroids, where both triamcinolone suspensions and dexamethasone implants show close to no reduction in effectiveness [58, 59]. This significantly diminishes the attractiveness of vitrectomy for pre-retinal hemorrhages in patients where the use of intravitreal anti-VEGF treatment should remain a viable option and the risk of further complications due to the remaining vitreous is marginal. The prime example is retinal vein occlusions.

Other Options

Observation, Nd:YAG membranotomy, and vitrectomy are the most common approaches to deal with pre-retinal hemorrhages. However, sometimes these treatment approaches are not feasible. For example, in infants, an early clearing to prevent amblyopia is desired excluding observation; a pediatric vitrectomy on the other hand proves often challenging, and bilateral cases require sequential vitrectomies of both eyes within a few days to prevent a monocular occlusion amblyopia. For such cases the combination of intravitreal recombinant tissue plasminogen activator (rtPA) and gas might be an option. Two pediatric patients with a bilateral pre-retinal hemorrhage after a non-accidental trauma responded well to repeated intravitreal injections of 25 μg rtPA and 0.25 mL of SF6 gas. The injections were continued weekly until the hemorrhage had cleared (three injections in all eyes). [5] In adult diabetics ($n = 5$), a similar series on a single dose of intravitreal rtPA (0.1 mL, 50 μg) and subsequent SF6 gas demonstrated complete reabsorption after 1 month. Subsequently the vitreous remained clear throughout the 6-month follow-up. [60] The concept was taken further by another group that treated seven diabetic eyes with a combination of Nd:YAG membranotomy, intravitreal rtPA(0.1 mL, 25 μg), and 0.2 mL of C3F8 gas. Notably their outcome was similar not only to the other combinations of rtPA and gas but also to studies on Nd:YAG membranotomy alone. [61] In another small case series, the combination of a single dose of bevacizumab with 0.2–0.3 mL of C3F8 gas also resulted in a resolution of the blood within a month, without the potentially increased risk of rebleeding when using rtPA. [62] In short, the combination of various treatment modalities is possible; if this is truly better than either conventional monotherapy or mere observation is, however, questionable. Thus, these approaches should be reserved for selected cases.

Conclusion

The main treatment options for pre-retinal and sub-ILM hemorrhages are observation, Nd:YAG membranotomy, and vitrectomy. The choice of treatment depends on the cause of the hemorrhage, the wish of the patient, and the comorbidities both ocular and extraocular. Generally, most small hemorrhages resolve spontaneously and without a sequel, but the resolution might take months. This needs to be addressed when discussing the treatment option with the patient. Given the favorable risk/benefit ratio, a Nd:YAG membranotomy should be considered in visually significant hemorrhages with a diameter greater than three disk diameters. This might also include proliferative diabetics if the visualization of the peripheral retina is sufficient to perform timely panretinal photocoagulation and the disease activity does not require urgent surgery. After all, a vitrectomy always remains an option.

References

1. Ko F, Knox DL. The ocular pathology of Terson's syndrome. Ophthalmology. 2010;117(7):1423–9.e2.
2. Zenoni S, Comi N, Fontana P. Individualised treatment of proliferative diabetic retinopathy: optimal surgical timing improves long-term outcomes. EPMA J. 2010;1(1):78–81.
3. Chanana B, Azad RV. Premacular subhyaloid haemorrhage in Eales' disease managed with Nd:YAG laser. Eye (Lond). 2009;23(7):1609–11.
4. Padhi TR, Das T, Rath S, Pradhan L, Sutar S, Panda KG, et al. Serial evaluation of retinal vascular changes in infants treated with intravitreal bevacizumab for aggressive posterior retinopathy of prematurity in zone I. Eye (Lond). 2016;30:392–9.
5. Conway MD, Peyman GA, Recasens M. Intravitreal tPA and SF6 promote clearing of premacular subhyaloid hemorrhages in shaken and battered baby syndrome. Ophthalmic Surg Lasers. 1999;30(6):435–41.
6. Chan CK, Ip MS, Vanveldhuisen PC, Oden NL, Scott IU, Tolentino MJ, et al. SCORE Study report #11: incidences of neovascular events in eyes with retinal vein occlusion. Ophthalmology. 2011;118(7):1364–72.
7. Cooper BA, Blinder KJ, Shah GK, Foster W, Leibole M. Femtosecond laser-induced premacular hemorrhage. Retina. 2004;24(5):812–4.
8. Alsulaiman SM, Alrushood AA, Almasaud J, Alzaaidi S, Alzahrani Y, Arevalo JF, et al. High-power handheld blue laser-induced maculopathy: the results of the King Khaled Eye Specialist Hospital Collaborative Retina Study Group. Ophthalmology. 2014;121(2):566–72.e1.
9. Sebag J. Age-related differences in the human vitreoretinal interface. Arch Ophthalmol. 1991;109(7):966–71.
10. Kuhn F, Morris R, Witherspoon CD, Mester V. Terson syndrome. Results of vitrectomy and the significance of vitreous hemorrhage in patients with subarachnoid hemorrhage. Ophthalmology. 1998;105(3):472–7.
11. Gardner HB. Do true preretinal (subhyaloid) hemorrhages occur in infants? Eur J Pediatr. 2012;171(3):597; author reply 9.
12. Emerson MV, Jakobs E, Green WR. Ocular autopsy and histopathologic features of child abuse. Ophthalmology. 2007;114(7):1384–94.
13. Meyer CH, Mennel S, Rodrigues EB, Schmidt JC. Is the location of valsalva hemorrhages submembranous or subhyaloidal? Am J Ophthalmol. 2006;141(1):231; author reply 2.
14. Kwok AK, Lai TY, Chan NR. Epiretinal membrane formation with internal limiting membrane wrinkling after Nd:YAG laser membranotomy in valsalva retinopathy. Am J Ophthalmol. 2003;136(4):763–6.
15. Shukla D, Naresh KB, Kim R. Optical coherence tomography findings in valsalva retinopathy. Am J Ophthalmol. 2005;140(1):134–6.
16. Matonti F, Donadieu V, Hoffart L, Dornadin A, Nadeau S, Roux S, et al. [Early treatment with Nd:YAG laser for valsalva retinopathy: results of five cases and literature review]. J Fr Ophtalmol. 2013;36(7):604–9.
17. Stiebel-Kalish H, Turtel LS, Kupersmith MJ. The natural history of nontraumatic subarachnoid hemorrhage-related intraocular hemorrhages. Retina. 2004;24(1):36–40.
18. Schultz PN, Sobol WM, Weingeist TA. Long-term visual outcome in Terson syndrome. Ophthalmology. 1991;98(12):1814–9.
19. Skevas C, Czorlich P, Knospe V, Stemplewitz B, Richard G, Westphal M, et al. Terson's syndrome–rate and surgical approach in patients with subarachnoid hemorrhage: a prospective interdisciplinary study. Ophthalmology. 2014;121(8):1628–33.
20. Szelog JT, Lally DR, Heier JS. Natural history of Valsalva-induced subhyaloid hemorrhage. JAMA Ophthalmol. 2015;133(2):e143268.

21. Gillies A, Lahav M. Absorption of retinal and subretinal hemorrhages. Ann Ophthalmol. 1983;15(11):1068–74.
22. Maar N, Tittl M, Ergun E, Stur M. [Results of fundus perimetry after resorbed premacular hemorrhages under the internal limiting membrane in 10 patients]. Klin Monbl Augenheilkd. 2000;217(5):269-73.
23. De Maeyer K, Van Ginderdeuren R, Postelmans L, Stalmans P, Van Calster J. Sub-inner limiting membrane haemorrhage: causes and treatment with vitrectomy. Br J Ophthalmol. 2007;91(7):869–72.
24. El-Bradey MH, Cheng L, Bartsch DU, Niessman M, El-Musharaf A, Freeman WR. The effect of prinomastat (AG3340), a potent inhibitor of matrix metalloproteinase, on a new animal model of epiretinal membrane. Retina. 2004;24(5):783–9.
25. Kono T, Kohno T, Inomata H. Epiretinal membrane formation. Light and electron microscopic study in an experimental rabbit model. Arch Ophthalmol. 1995;113(3):359–63.
26. Yazici AT, Alagoz N, Celik HU, Bozkurt E, Alagoz C, Cakir M, et al. Idiopathic and secondary epiretinal membranes: do they differ in terms of morphology? An optical coherence tomography-based study. Retina. 2011;31(4):779–84.
27. Rubowitz A, Desai U. Nontraumatic macular holes associated with Terson syndrome. Retina. 2006;26(2):230–2.
28. Xie ZG, Yu SQ, Chen X, Zhu J, Chen F. Macular hole secondary to valsalva retinopathy after doing push-up exercise. BMC Ophthalmol. 2014;14:98.
29. AlHarkan DH, Kahtani ES, Gikandi PW, Abu El-Asrar AM. Vitreous hemorrhage in pediatric age group. J Ophthalmol. 2014;2014:497083.
30. Goldenberg DT, Wu D, Capone A Jr, Drenser KA, Trese MT. Nonaccidental trauma and peripheral retinal nonperfusion. Ophthalmology. 2010;117(3):561–6.
31. Spirn MJ, Lynn MJ, Hubbard GB III. Vitreous hemorrhage in children. Ophthalmology. 2006;113(5):848–52.
32. Fechner PU. [Premacular hemorrhage: a new indication for argon-laser-therapy (author's transl)]. Klin Monbl Augenheilkd. 1980;177(4):502–5.
33. Khairallah M, Ladjimi A, Messaoud R, Ben Yahia S, Hmidi K, Jenzeri S. Retinal venous macroaneurysm associated with premacular hemorrhage. Ophthalmic Surg Lasers. 1999;30(3):226–8.
34. Sahu DK, Namperumalsamy P, Kim R, Ravindran RD. Argon laser treatment for premacular hemorrhage. Retina. 1998;18(1):79–82.
35. Faulborn J. Behandlung einer diabetischen pramakularen Blutung mit dem Q-switched Neodym:YAG laser. Spektrum Augenheilkd. 1988;2:33–5.
36. Ulbig MW, Mangouritsas G, Rothbacher HH, Hamilton AM, McHugh JD. Long-term results after drainage of premacular subhyaloid hemorrhage into the vitreous with a pulsed Nd:YAG laser. Arch Ophthalmol. 1998;116(11):1465–9.
37. Durukan AH, Kerimoglu H, Erdurman C, Demirel A, Karagul S. Long-term results of Nd:YAG laser treatment for premacular subhyaloid haemorrhage owing to Valsalva retinopathy. Eye (Lond). 2008;22(2):214–8.
38. Raymond LA. Neodymium:YAG laser treatment for hemorrhages under the internal limiting membrane and posterior hyaloid face in the macula. Ophthalmology. 1995;102(3):406–11.
39. Bonner RF, Meyers SM, Gaasterland DE. Threshold for retinal damage associated with the use of high-power neodymium-YAG lasers in the vitreous. Am J Ophthalmol. 1983;96(2):153–9.
40. Zou M, Gao S, Zhang J, Zhang M. Persistent unsealed internal limiting membrane after Nd:YAG laser treatment for valsalva retinopathy. BMC Ophthalmol. 2013;13:15.
41. Ezra E, Dowler JG, Burgess F, Sehmi K, Hamilton PA. Identifying maculopathy after neodymium: YAG membranotomy for dense diabetic premacular hemorrhage. Ophthalmology. 1996;103(10):1568–74.
42. Rizzo S, Pellegrini G, Benocci F, Belting C, Baicchi U, Vispi M. Autologous plasmin for pharmacologic vitreolysis prepared 1 hour before surgery. Retina. 2006;26(7):792–6.
43. Velikay M, Datlinger P, Stolba U, Wedrich A, Binder S, Hausmann N. Retinal detachment with severe proliferative vitreoretinopathy in Terson syndrome. Ophthalmology. 1994;101(1):35–7.
44. Mansour A. Nd:YAG laser photodisruption of hemorrhagic detachment of the internal limiting membrane. Am J Ophthalmol. 1989;107(5):566–8.
45. Pichi F, Ciardella AP, Torrazza C, Morara M, Scano G, Mattana G, et al. A spectral-domain optical coherence tomography description of ND: YAG laser hyaloidotomy in premacular subhyaloid hemorrhage. Retina. 2012;32(4):861–2.
46. O'Hanley GP, Canny CL. Diabetic dense premacular hemorrhage. A possible indication for prompt vitrectomy. Ophthalmology. 1985;92(4):507–11.
47. Frizzell RT, Kuhn F, Morris R, Quinn C, Fisher WS III. Screening for ocular hemorrhages in patients with ruptured cerebral aneurysms: a prospective study of 99 patients. Neurosurgery. 1997;41(3):529–33; discussion 533–4
48. Fountas KN, Kapsalaki EZ, Lee GP, Machinis TG, Grigorian AA, Robinson JS, et al. Terson hemorrhage in patients suffering aneurysmal subarachnoid hemorrhage: predisposing factors and prognostic significance. J Neurosurg. 2008;109(3):439–44.
49. Clarkson JG, Flynn HW Jr, Daily MJ. Vitrectomy in Terson's syndrome. Am J Ophthalmol. 1980;90(4):549–52.
50. Early vitrectomy for severe vitreous hemorrhage in diabetic retinopathy. Four-year results of a randomized trial: Diabetic Retinopathy Vitrectomy Study Report 5. Arch Ophthalmol. 1990;108(7):958–64.
51. Li X, Jiang Y, Ye C, Li C. [Timing of vitrectomy for proliferative diabetic retinopathy in cases with

type II diabetes mellitus]. Zhonghua Yan Ke Za Zhi. 1999;35(2):116–8.
52. West JF, Gregor ZJ. Fibrovascular ingrowth and recurrent haemorrhage following diabetic vitrectomy. Br J Ophthalmol. 2000;84(8):822–5.
53. Novak MA, Rice TA, Michels RG, Auer C. Vitreous hemorrhage after vitrectomy for diabetic retinopathy. Ophthalmology. 1984;91(12):1485–9.
54. Yang CM. Surgical treatment for diabetic retinopathy: 5-year experience. J Formos Med Assoc. 1998;97(7):477–84.
55. Yeh PT, Yang CM, Yang CH. Distribution, reabsorption, and complications of preretinal blood under silicone oil after vitrectomy for severe proliferative diabetic retinopathy. Eye (Lond). 2012;26(4):601–8.
56. Yeh PT, Yang CM, Lin YC, Chen MS, Yang CH. Bevacizumab pretreatment in vitrectomy with silicone oil for severe diabetic retinopathy. Retina. 2009;29(6):768–74.
57. Moisseiev E, Waisbourd M, Ben-Artsi E, Levinger E, Barak A, Daniels T, et al. Pharmacokinetics of bevacizumab after topical and intravitreal administration in human eyes. Graefes Arch Clin Exp Ophthalmol. 2014;252(2):331–7.
58. Watanabe A, Tsuzuki A, Arai K, Gekka T, Kohzaki K, Tsuneoka H. Efficacy of intravitreal triamcinolone acetonide for diabetic macular edema after vitrectomy. J Ocul Pharmacol Ther. 2016;32:38–43.
59. Medeiros MD, Alkabes M, Navarro R, Garcia-Arumi J, Mateo C, Corcostegui B. Dexamethasone intravitreal implant in vitrectomized versus nonvitrectomized eyes for treatment of patients with persistent diabetic macular edema. J Ocul Pharmacol Ther. 2014;30(9):709–16.
60. Yang CM, Chen MS. Tissue plasminogen activator and gas for diabetic premacular hemorrhage. Am J Ophthalmol. 2000;129(3):393–4.
61. Chung J, Park YH, Lee YC. The effect of Nd:YAG laser membranotomy and intravitreal tissue plasminogen activator with gas on massive diabetic premacular hemorrhage. Ophthalmic Surg Lasers Imaging. 2008;39(2):114–20.
62. Shih CW, Yang CM, Chen MS, Wang TJ. Intravitreal injection of bevacizumab and gas for diabetic premacular hemorrhage with active fibrovascular proliferation. Graefes Arch Clin Exp Ophthalmol. 2008;246(11):1547–51.

Surgical Treatment of Massive Subretinal Hemorrhage

7

Peter Szurman and Kai Januschowski

Indication

The treatment of age-related macular degeneration (AMD) has changed for the better in the last decade, and new treatment options have been and are discovered recently, with most of them being pharmacological. The intravitreal pharmacotherapy as the new treatment of choice has mostly replaced the surgical approach. Today an indication for surgery exists only for certain forms of hemorrhagic choroidal neovascularization (CNV) with a significant subretinal hemorrhage. In such cases the optimal treatment option is still discussed.

Small- and medium-sized subretinal bleedings are associated with a better visual prognosis and are generally not operated. In most cases a simple displacement of the subretinal blood away from the central part of the retina toward the periphery followed by pharmacological treatment of the neovascular membrane is sufficient [1].

In cases of massive hemorrhages with a high blood volume that are not limited to the vascular arcades or in association with a hemorrhagic retinal detachment, the success of displacing the bleeding is rather questionable [2]. Lytic therapy hardly removes all the hemorrhage from the center, even if combined with air or gas tamponades. Failure to start an adequate therapy leads to a dramatic loss of best corrected visual acuity (BCVA) and visual field function (Fig. 7.1).

Fortunately the development of the surgical techniques has advanced over the last years providing patients with severe cases of subretinal mass hemorrhages with good albeit not excellent treatment options. Subretinal surgery still has an indication in cases of mentioned massive hemorrhages that are not within the vascular arcades and hemorrhagic retinal detachments, but the decision for or against surgery should always be based on the individual clinical situation.

Surgical Techniques of Subretinal Drainage

Subretinal Extraction of Membranes

Keeping in mind that removing the hemorrhage is the symptomatic treatment of a complication caused by a neovascular membrane, it is not surprising that results of only removing the bleeding were not convincing [3]. Treating the underlying cause by either intravitreal pharmacotherapy or extracting the membrane surgically should therefore always be considered.

De Juan and Machemer reported the successful surgical removal of CNV membranes as early

P. Szurman, M.D. (✉) · K. Januschowski, M.D.
Eye Clinic Sulzbach, Sulzbach/Saar, Germany

Center for ophthalmology, Eberhard-Karls University, Tuebingen, Germany
e-mail: Peter.Szurman@kksaar.de

L.-O. Hattenbach (ed.), *Management of Macular Hemorrhage*,
https://doi.org/10.1007/978-3-319-65877-3_7

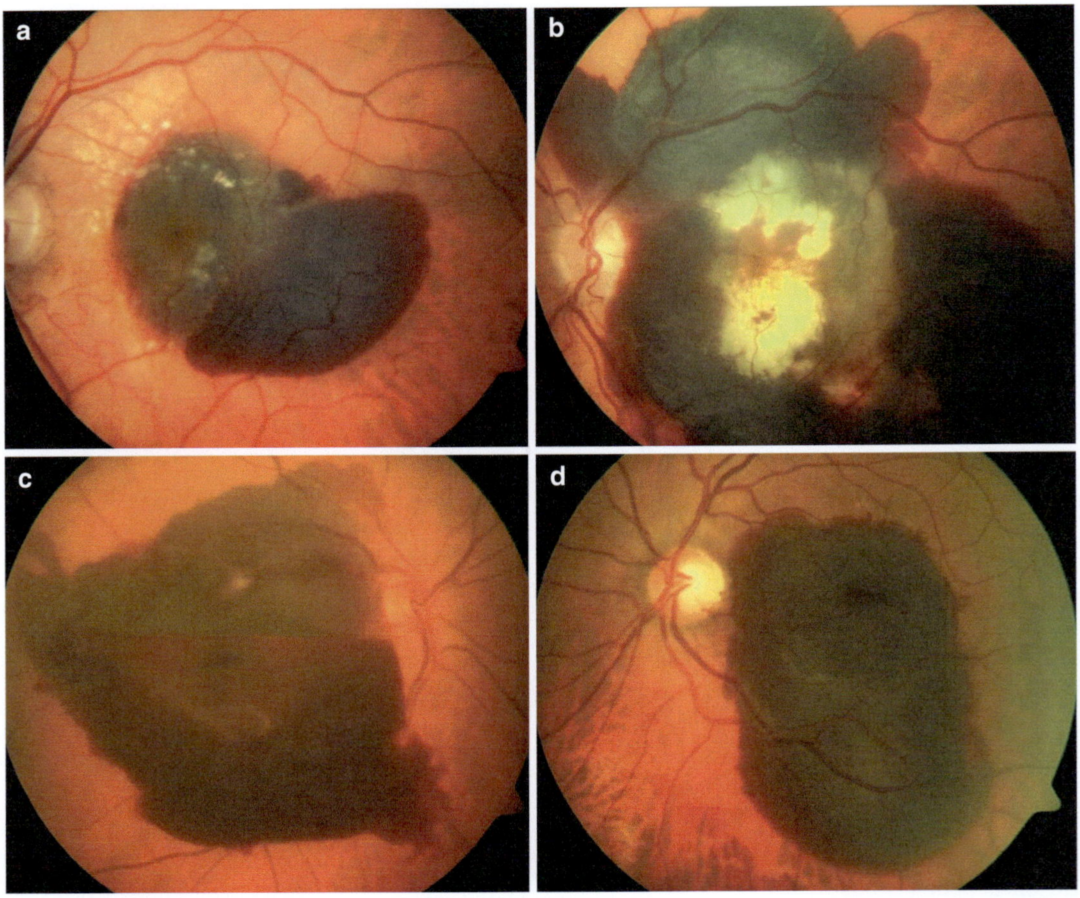

Fig. 7.1 Fundus of a fresh subretinal mass hemorrhage with retrohyaloidal parts in a patient (**a-d**) with exudative AMD

as 1988 [4]. Improving the surgical technique, this procedure became popular quick. The membrane is removed via a small retinotomy in the temporal raphe or in the vicinity of the vascular arcades [5]. While not exerting too extensive retinal trauma, the clotted blood including the causing membrane can be removed as a whole through this opening resulting in transient visual improvement but unfortunately in only few cases. This improvement in BCVA usually only lasts for a limited amount of months due to the extensive RPE defect. Moreover the blood and fibrin clot adheres to the RPE causing a greater extension of the RPE defect after extraction. The Submacular Surgery Trial (SST) compared the development of BCVA of surgically treated AMD patients to a group of patients that were only observed [6]. Hemorrhagic CNV was evaluated as a separate group (SST group B) and failed to show a benefit when compared with the natural course. Because of the resulting RPE defect, a progredient visual loss was reported in the first year of the study in contrast to patients treated with photocoagulation. Patients who were only observed even showed a slight long-term improvement. This was not the case for surgically treated patients.

Even though membrane extraction in cases of massive subretinal hemorrhage reduces the risk of severe visual impairment, only 20% of treated patients had an increase of BCVA of more than two lines, while 56% lost two lines or more [7]. An additional injection with rTPA did not improve these results. It has to be mentioned that the SST results were generally poor and hardly any patients profited from surgery, while surgical complications mostly caused by the retinotomies were quite relevant.

Interestingly another retrospective study analyzing 42 eyes showed different results: After removal of the CNV membrane and the subretinal hemorrhage, patients had a significantly better visual outcome than a group with patients where the blood was displaced by injection of an air bubble into the vitreous cavity. The latter group had satisfying short-term results that did not last for a longer follow-up due to further evolution of the CNV membrane. These results were obviously reported before the area of anti-VEGF injections and would probably be different today [8].

Translocation of the Macula with 360° Retinotomy

We have learned from the SST that an intact RPE is essential for a long-term BCVA stabilization and that removal of the blood clot with the CNV membrane basically damages the RPE underlying the macula.

Translocating the macula using a 360° retinotomy (Fig. 7.2) was the first approach acknowledging this. Again, Machemer and Steinhorst pioneered in 1993 and introduced the concept of moving the macula to a healthy RPE and laid the foundations of the nowadays most important surgical technique in submacular surgery for AMD [9]. After a pars plana vitrectomy (ppV), the retina is artificially detached with subretinal irrigation, mobilized with a 360° retinotomy, and folded in order to create enough space to remove even large subretinal bleedings including the causative CNV membrane. At the time that the first three cases were published, no treatment options existed for patients with large submacular hemorrhages. Eckardt et al. significantly improved the resulting strabologic problems by counterrotation of the ocular muscles [10]. Later on, Wong et al. could confirm that especially eyes with large bleedings can potentially benefit from macular translocation with 360° retinotomy, because the removal of the blood is facilitated by folding the retina [11]. Nevertheless, clinical experience has taught us that the blood-fibrin clot removal with the cutter is not easy because during the cutting process the clot is often detached from the instrument and needs to be aspirated again. Reducing the cutter and aspiration rate usually helps to resolve the hemorrhage entirely.

Other studies have analyzed the outcome of subretinal surgery on CNV with mass subretinal hemorrhage separately and could show that these patients seem to benefit from macular translocation with 360° retinotomy [12]. In the first prospective study including 90 patients with hemorrhagic CNV, of whom 26 had a significant bleeding, an increase of four letters was reported for patients with a large bleeding during the first year. Compared to classic CNV without

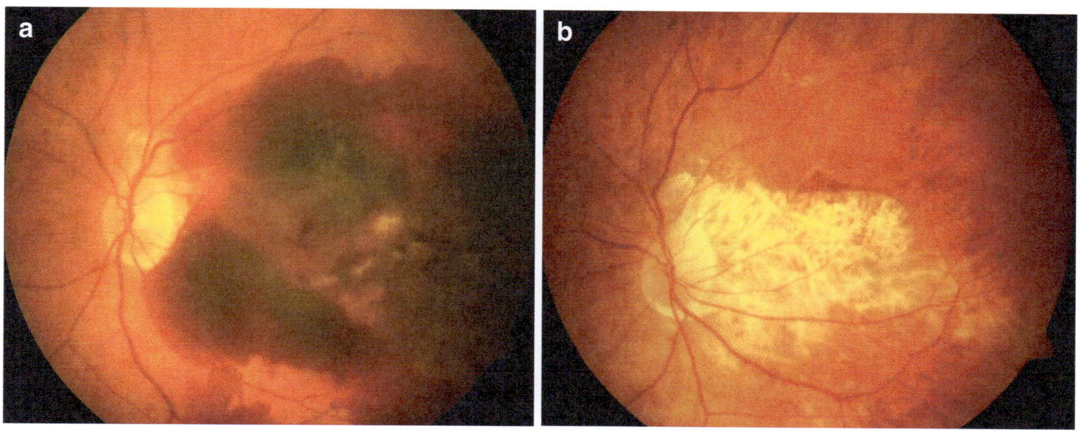

Fig. 7.2 Fundus of a patient with submacular hemorrhage before (**a**) and after (**b**) macular translocation

bleeding (increase of two lines), these results are worse but better compared to occult CNV without bleeding (loss of 2.5 lines). An explanation for this finding was discussed to be the fact that patients with classic CNV usually develop symptoms earlier than patients with occult CNV and therefore received surgical treatment earlier [13]. Thirty percent of patients with hemorrhagic CNV were reported to have an increase in BCVA of three lines. After a 5-year follow-up period, this improvement in BCVA could be sustained [14]. Unfortunately long-existing and especially large hemorrhages are problematic because the RPE is impacted over a large area thus limiting options of macular translocation. In the mentioned study, the fovea had to be relocated over an area of atrophy in spite of maximal rotation in nine eyes. Most of them had a hemorrhagic CNV.

Macular translocation usually only stabilizes BCVA even though some patients have a quite remarkable functional outcome. This is explained by the fact that especially patients with complications have a severe functional loss: Eyes with hemorrhagic CNV were reported to have a 19% rate of retinal detachment after surgery during the first year and 23% after 3 years, respectively. Another limiting factor of invasive submacular surgical procedures in the treatment of wet AMD is the development of a proliferative vitreoretinopathy (PVR) reaction that should not be underestimated.

Translocation of the Choroid and Retinal Pigment Epithelium

Due to the high rate of PVR and the associated strabologic problems of the macular translocation, the concept of translocating a patch of choroid and RPE was developed: A block excision of the RPE, Bruch's membrane, and choroid at the equator is performed, and this patch is placed under the macula after removal of the hemorrhage and CNV membrane [15, 16]. Because no strabologic problems resulting from translocation of the fovea occurre, no additional counter-rotation of the ocular muscles is necessary.

Two approaches exist today to obtain a RPE-choroid patch: The smaller one consists of translocating a patch using a medium-sized retinotomy at the superior vascular arcade or the temporal raphe without folding the retina [15]. Advantages are the minimal invasiveness of the procedure and the shorter operation time; the disadvantages are size of the patch, harder relocation of the patch under the fovea, a more difficult removal of the clotted blood, and restricted possibilities of coagulating new occurring bleedings during surgery. Therefore this approach is problematic in cases of massive hemorrhage.

As an alternative a 180° retinotomy can be performed that allows folding the retina, removing the blood under controlled circumstances and generating larger patches of RPE and choroid [16] (Fig. 7.3). This is especially important

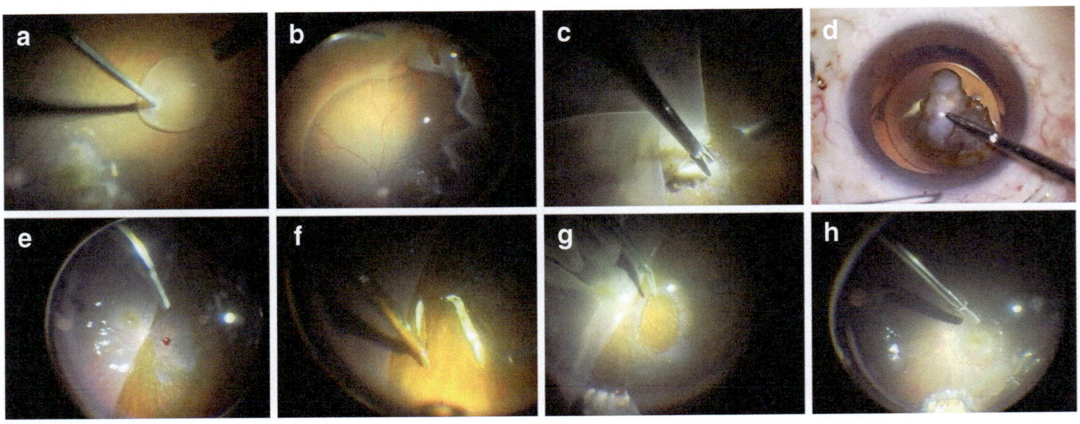

Fig. 7.3 Intraoperative picture: After mobilization of the retina (**a**, **b**), the membrane is extracted (**c**, **d**). Later on an RPE-choroid patch in the middle periphery (**e**) is and transferred under the macula (**f–h**)

regarding the fact that every transplant shows shrinkage at the edges over time. This results in dysfunction of smaller autologous transplants (Fig. 7.4). The easy access to the subretinal space not only allows easy removal of the CNV membrane but also of large submacular hemorrhages. Therefore, this option is the more promising one in cases of extensive subretinal bleedings. One small case series could even show an increase to a medium BCVA of 0.4 [15, 17]; another study including 21 patients had an improvement in 13 eyes, a stabilization in 2 eyes, and a deterioration in 6 eyes, despite complete removal of the hemorrhage [16]. In a recent study, 17 eyes with a sustained improvement of BCVA after 1 year of 2 lines were reported, but none of the eyes regained their reading BCVA [18]. Van Zeeburg et al. could report at least 5% of eyes that sustained or regained the ability to read in the study with the longest follow-up period (Figs. 7.5 and 7.6) [19].

Hemorrhagic lesions have a significantly worse outcome after translocation of the choroid and retinal pigment epithelium than nonhemorrhagic lesions [20], but the reduced visual prognosis is a general problem: A vascular supply of the patch by subfoveal vasculature makes a stabilization generally possible and is observed in most of the cases. But because revascularization takes up to 3 weeks, functional outcome is limited to the ischemic period (Fig. 7.6) [15]. Revascularization can be accelerated by surgically stimulating Bruch's membrane, but this only shortens the ischemic time interval. Because of this systematic problem, further improvement options of this procedure are limited (Fig. 7.7).

Looking at the complication rate, translocation of the choroid and retinal pigment epithelium has also failed to meet the expectations because it is only slightly better than the complication rate

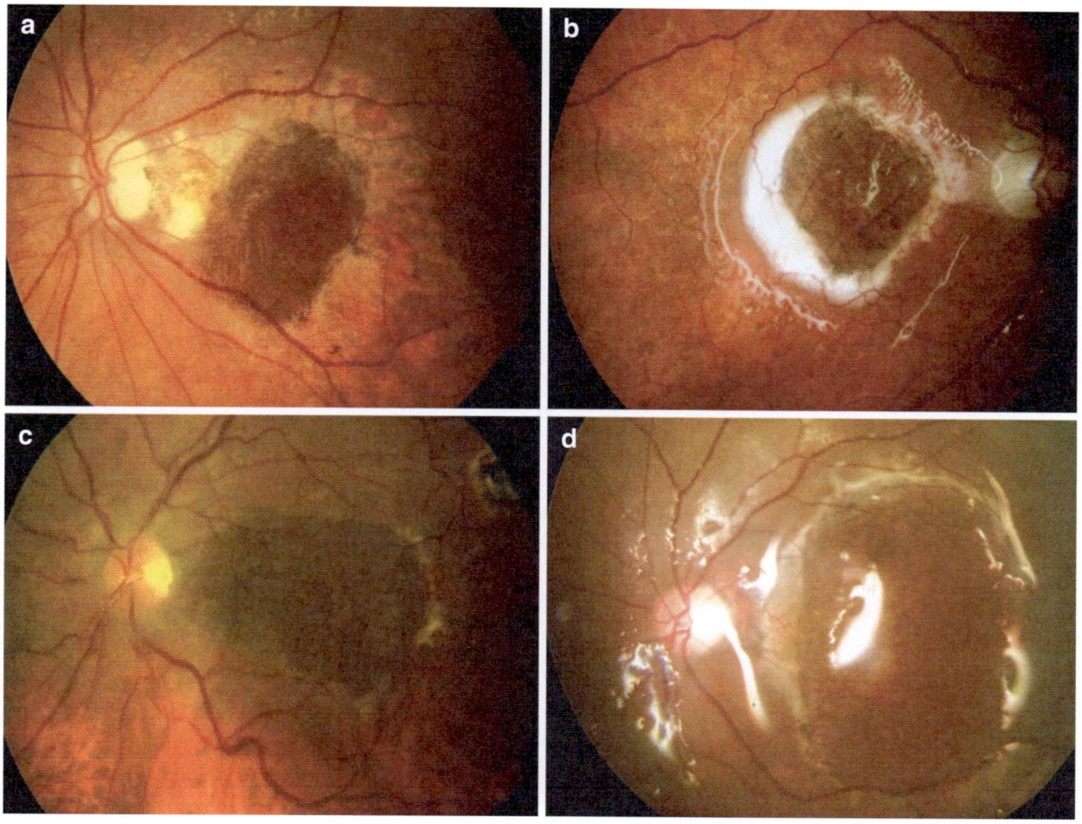

Fig. 7.4 Different postoperative findings after a RPE-choroid patch (**a-d**). A larger intraoperative approach permits the generation of larger transplants. An important point considering the shrinkage of the transplants

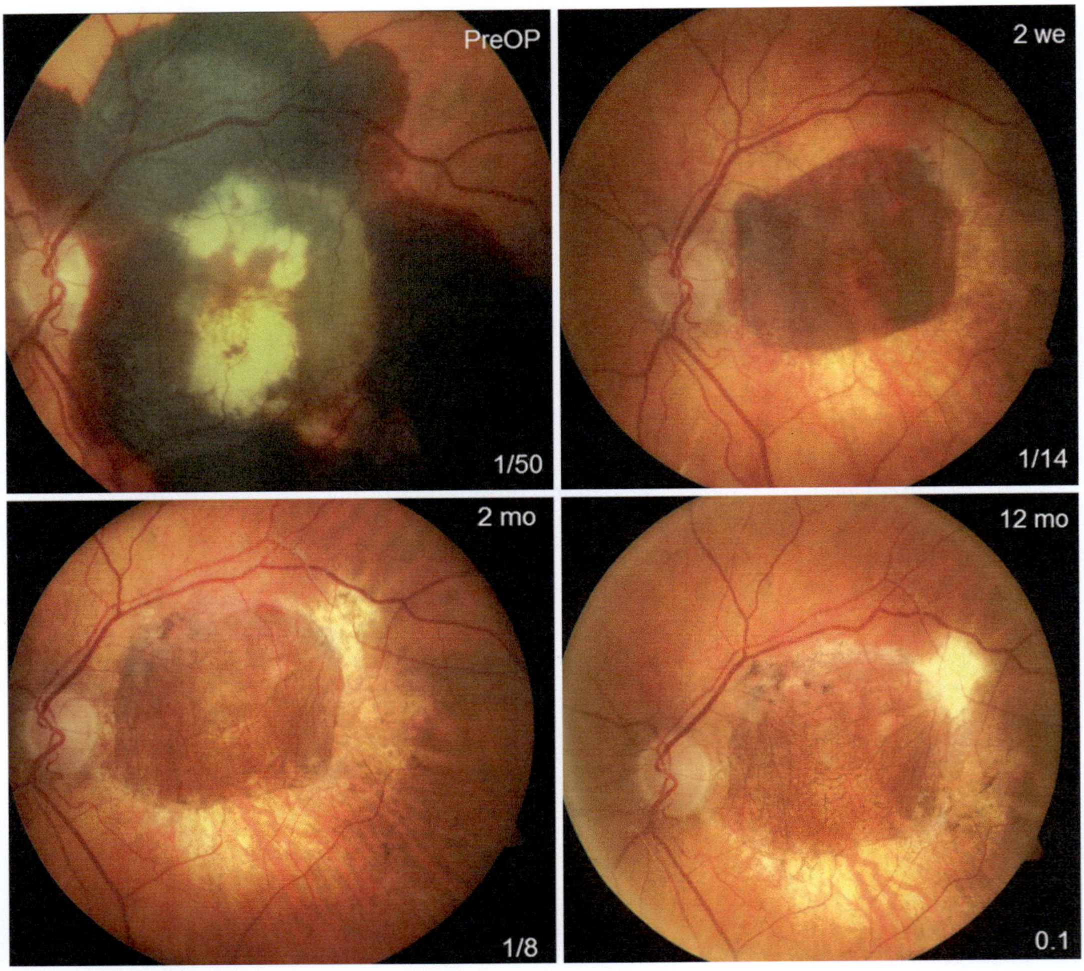

Fig. 7.5 Development of BCVA and RPE-choroid patch over time

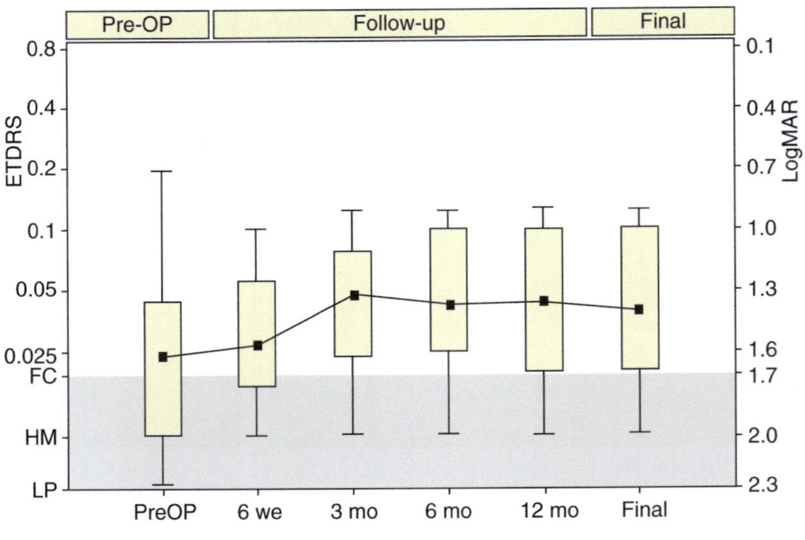

Fig. 7.6 Box plot of BCVA (LogMAR) over 12 months. Seventeen eyes after RPE-choroid patch were included

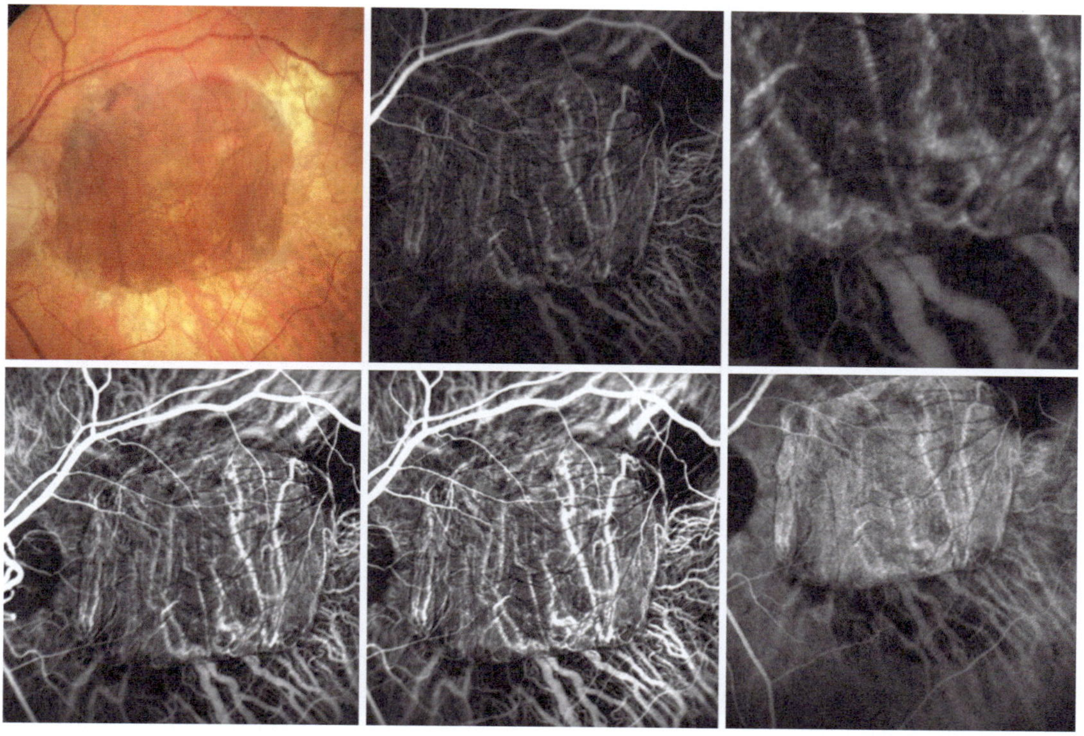

Fig. 7.7 Fundus and ICG angiography 2 months after RPE-choroid patch. The vascular connection is clearly demonstrated at different time points of the examination

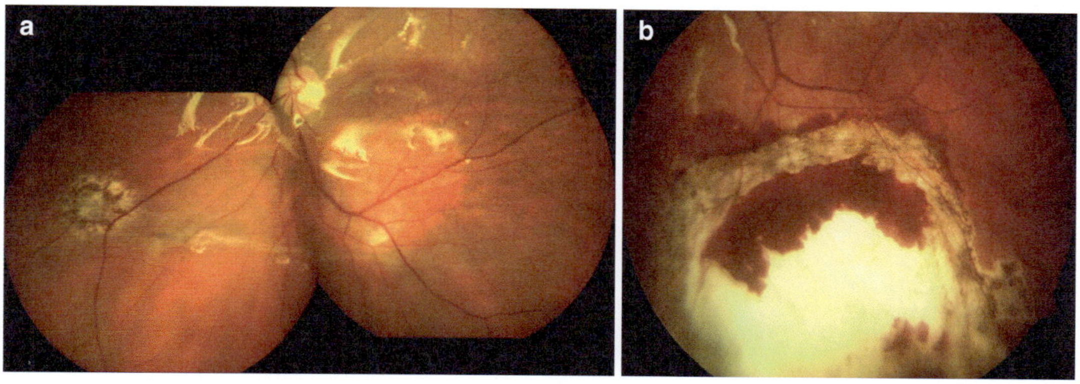

Fig. 7.8 Fundus 6 months after surgery. PVR traction (**a**) and late bleeding from the excision site (**b**) are also common postoperative complications

of macular translocation: 24% of patients had a PVR originating at the retinotomy or patch excision sites (Fig. 7.8) [18]. The subretinal tractions often require a continuous tamponade with silicone oil. This is supported by other studies reporting complication rates between 10 and 31% [15, 19].

Subretinal Drainage

In general less invasive procedures with smaller retinotomies do not permit the removal of larger blood clots. Therefore, in order to choose a less invasive procedure, one must resolve or partly resolve the mass hemorrhage. If this is successful, then even larger amounts of blood can be removed entirely via a small retinotomy. Kamei et al. first suggested this approach that was later on optimized by Oshima et al. [21, 22]. Both authors used rTPA to resolve the clotting and then mechanically kneaded the blood through a small retinotomy using a PFCL bubble (Fig. 7.9). Using rTPA was described in the SST as well [6], but the idea of using a PFCL bubble to really express the hemorrhage without too much mechanical manipulation was new [21] and showed that 16 out of 22 eyes reached a BCVA of 0.2 or better [5]. Oshima optimized the technique by injecting rTPA 12–24 h before performing the ppV [22] and funduscopically verifying that the blood clot was resolved. During the second procedure, the blood was moved to the middle periphery and drained through one or two retinotomies. After a gas exchange, the patient was placed in the prone position. In his study, Oshima included eight eyes with an extensive hemorrhage reaching the periphery and could report a successful drainage in all cases; seven eyes reached a BCVA up to 0.32 without surgical complications. Considering the severity of the preoperative conditions, this operative procedure seems to be very promising, although it has to be mentioned that in this Japanese study population more than half of the eyes had a polypoidal vasculopathy that is known to have a better prognosis per se.

Moreover, the dose of 5 µg rTPA, as described by Oshima, is in many cases not sufficient to entirely resolve a mass hemorrhage. In our experience 100 µg rTPA 1 day before surgery is a better option. This equals an intravitreal concentration of about 20 µg/mL and is not retinotoxic. Lueke et al. reported a concentration of 60 µg/mL to be toxic in the pseudo-in vivo model of an isolated vertebrate retina [23]. A dose of at least 20 µg/mL is mandatory in clinical experience to resolve the clot. As suggested by Oshima et al., resolution of the blood clot should be verified funduscopically, because in some cases a second injection of rTPA is necessary. Only after a verified resolution of the clot should a 23 gauge pars plana vitrectomy (ppV) inducing a posterior vitreous detachment be performed. Instead of using a PCFL bubble, it is also possible to use a fine 41 gauge needle (DORC, Rotterdam) to subretinally inject balanced salt solution and irrigate the hemorrhage. Using a juxtamacular retinotomy, the blood can be drained into the vitreous cavity; remaining parts of the bleeding can then be removed with a PFCL bubble and gentle movements of the eye (Fig. 7.10). The small irrigation retinotomy with the 41 gauge needle is self-sealing, and only the juxtamacular drainage site should be sealed with retinal photocoagulation. At the end of the procedure, a short-acting intravitreal air tamponade is sufficient because no pneumatic displacement of

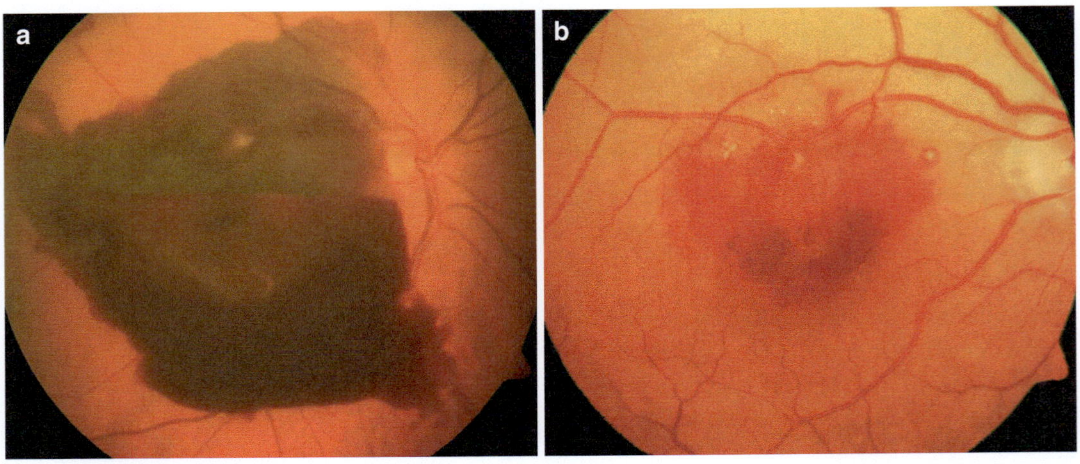

Fig. 7.9 Preoperative (**a**) and (**b**) postoperative situation after subretinal drainage in a patient with mass hemorrhage in wet AMD

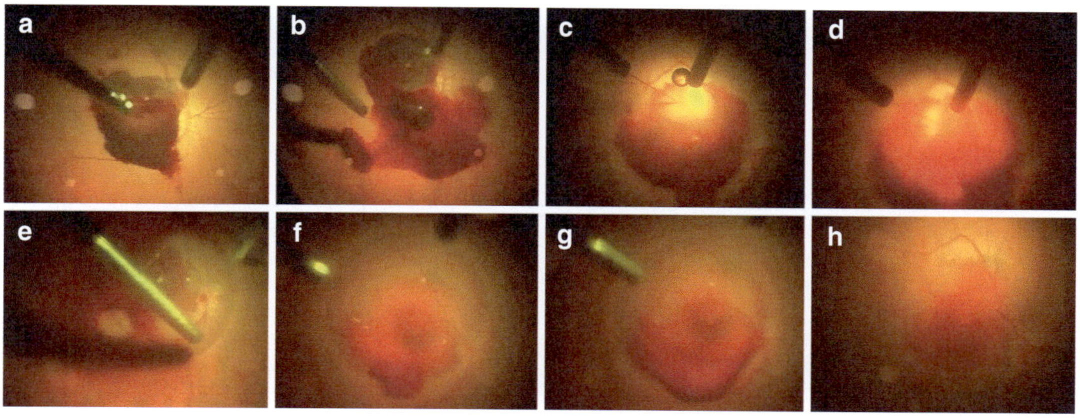

Fig. 7.10 Intraoperative situation during subretinal drainage. rTPA in this case was injected 24 h prior and the bleeding has resolved (**a**). Irrigation is performed with a 41 gauge needle, and the bleeding is drained via an additional retinotomy (**b-d**). Remaining blood can be kneaded away using a PFCL bubble (**e-g**). Complete removal of the subretinal hemorrhage is possible (**h**)

Table 7.1 Complications after subretinal drainage ($n = 21$)

Extrafoveal rem. hemorrhage	38% [8]
Retinal detachment	5% [1]
PVR	–
Secondary ppV	5% [1]
Vitreous hemorrhage	24% [5]

remaining blood is necessary (Video unter www.augenklinik-sulzbach.de). In an analysis of 21 eyes with subretinal drainage after mass hemorrhage, an increase in BCVA of 8 lines was observed with a median increase of 0.025–0.16. Six eyes even reached reading BCVA or better [18]. Using this rather minimal invasive technique, the rate of complications is rather low, no PVR reaction was observed, and a second surgery was only necessary in one case (Table 7.1) [18]. This approach avoids damage to the RPE by surgically removing the CNV membrane. Further treatment with anti-VEGF and close follow-up of the patient every 4–8 weeks may be necessary [24, 25].

The controversy about the use of rTPA is still ongoing [26]. The question whether rTPA diffuses into the subretinal space is imminent with rPTA having a molecular weight of about 65 kDa. In a rabbit model, no diffusion into the subretinal space was reported [27], whereas diffusion was reported indeed in a porcine model [28]. In the event of a massive subretinal hemorrhage, microlesions are likely to be present thus facilitating diffusion into the subretinal space [29], although interindividual differences may play an important role. Recently the use of third-generation thrombolytic tenecteplase has been reported to penetrate the retina; therefore this might be another interesting treatment option in the future [30].

Conclusion

Massive subretinal hemorrhage in patients with exudative AMD is associated with a negative visual prognosis. These cases cannot be treated with simple intravitreal rTPA and gas injection and should be approached surgically. It should always be considered that apart from removing the hemorrhage, treatment of the hemorrhagic CNV is essential. Possible treatment options are macular translocation in severe cases where the second eye is involved or a RPE and choroidal translocation if only one eye is involved to prevent strabologic problems.

A much safer procedure with less complications and better visual outcome is the two-step approach of injecting rTPA to resolve the clot and performing a ppV subretinal drainage via a small retinotomy later on.

References

1. Ritzau-Tondrow U, Baraki H, Hoerauf H. [Minimally invasive therapy of submacular hemorrhage in exsudative age-related macular degeneration]. Ophthalmologe. 2012;109(7):670–5.
2. Hassan AS, Johnson MW, Schneiderman TE, Regillo CD, Tornambe PE, Poliner LS, et al. Management of submacular hemorrhage with intravitreous tissue plasminogen activator injection and pneumatic displacement. Ophthalmology [Clinical Trial Multicenter Study]. 1999;106(10):1900–6; discussion 1906–7.
3. Vander JF. Tissue plasminogen activator irrigation to facilitate removal of subretinal hemorrhage during vitrectomy. Ophthalmic Surg [Case Reports]. 1992; 23(5):361–3.
4. de Juan E Jr, Machemer R. Vitreous surgery for hemorrhagic and fibrous complications of age-related macular degeneration. Am J Ophthalmol. [Case Reports Research Support, Non-U.S. Gov't Research Support, U.S. Gov't, P.H.S.]. 1988;105(1):25–9.
5. Thomas MA, Grand MG, Williams DF, Lee CM, Pesin SR, Lowe MA. Surgical management of subfoveal choroidal neovascularization. Ophthalmology. [Case Reports Research Support, Non-U.S. Gov't]. 1992;99(6):952–68; discussion 75–6.
6. Bressler NM, Bressler SB, Childs AL, Haller JA, Hawkins BS, Lewis H, et al. Surgery for hemorrhagic choroidal neovascular lesions of age-related macular degeneration: ophthalmic findings: SST report no. 13. Ophthalmology. [Clinical Trial Multicenter Study Randomized Controlled Trial Research Support, U.S. Gov't, P.H.S.]. 2004;111(11):1993–2006.
7. Falkner CI, Leitich H, Frommlet F, Bauer P, Binder S. The end of submacular surgery for age-related macular degeneration? A meta-analysis. Graefes Arch Clin Exp Ophthalmol [Meta-Analysis]. 2007;245(4): 490–501.
8. Thompson JT, Sjaarda RN. Vitrectomy for the treatment of submacular hemorrhages from macular degeneration: a comparison of submacular hemorrhage/membrane removal and submacular tissue plasminogen activator-assisted pneumatic displacement. Trans Am Ophthalmol Soc [Comparative Study Evaluation Studies]. 2005;103:98–107; discussion.
9. Machemer R, Steinhorst UH. Retinal separation, retinotomy, and macular relocation: II. A surgical approach for age-related macular degeneration? Graefes Arch Clin Exp Ophthalmol [Case Reports Research Support, Non-U.S. Gov't]. 1993;231(11):635–41.
10. Eckardt C, Eckardt U, Conrad HG. Macular rotation with and without counter-rotation of the globe in patients with age-related macular degeneration. Graefes Arch Clin Exp Ophthalmol [Comparative Study]. 1999;237(4):313–25.
11. Wong D, Stanga P, Briggs M, Lenfestey P, Lancaster E, Li KK, et al. Case selection in macular relocation surgery for age related macular degeneration. Br J Ophthalmol [Research Support, Non-U.S. Gov't]. 2004;88(2):186–90.
12. Pertile G, Claes C. Macular translocation with 360 degree retinotomy for management of age-related macular degeneration with subfoveal choroidal neovascularization. Am J Ophthalmol. 2002;134(4):560–5.
13. Aisenbrey S, Lafaut BA, Szurman P, Grisanti S, Luke C, Krott R, et al. Macular translocation with 360 degrees retinotomy for exudative age-related macular degeneration. Arch Ophthalmol. 2002;120(4):451–9.
14. Aisenbrey S, Bartz-Schmidt KU, Walter P, Hilgers RD, Ayertey H, Szurman P, et al. Long-term follow-up of macular translocation with 360 degrees retinotomy for exudative age-related macular degeneration. Arch Ophthalmol [Research Support, Non-U.S. Gov't]. 2007;125(10):1367–72.
15. Joussen AM, Heussen FM, Joeres S, Llacer H, Prinz B, Rohrschneider K, et al. Autologous translocation of the choroid and retinal pigment epithelium in age-related macular degeneration. Am J Ophthalmol [Research Support, Non-U.S. Gov't]. 2006;142(1):17–30.
16. van Meurs JC, Van Den Biesen PR. Autologous retinal pigment epithelium and choroid translocation in patients with exudative age-related macular degeneration: short-term follow-up. Am J Ophthalmol. 2003;136(4):688–95.
17. Gibran SK, Romano MR, Wong D. Perfluorocarbon liquid assisted large retinal epithelium patching in submacular hemorrhage secondary to age related macular degeneration. Graefes Arch Clin Exp Ophthalmol [Clinical Trial]. 2009;247(2):187–91.
18. Szurman P. [Subretinal surgery for massive hemorrhage]. Ophthalmologe. 2012;109(7):657–64.
19. van Zeeburg EJ, Maaijwee KJ, TO M, Heimann H, van Meurs JC. A free retinal pigment epithelium-choroid graft in patients with exudative age-related macular degeneration: results up to 7 years. Am J Ophthalmol [Research Support, Non-U.S. Gov't]. 2012;153(1):120–7e2.
20. Maaijwee K, Heimann H, Missotten T, Mulder P, Joussen A, van Meurs J. Retinal pigment epithelium and choroid translocation in patients with exudative age-related macular degeneration: long-term results. Graefes Arch Clin Exp Ophthalmol [Research Support, Non-U.S. Gov't]. 2007;245(11):1681–9.
21. Kamei M, Tano Y, Maeno T, Ikuno Y, Mitsuda H, Yuasa T. Surgical removal of submacular hemorrhage using tissue plasminogen activator and perfluorocarbon liquid. Am J Ophthalmol. 1996;121(3):267–75.
22. Oshima Y, Ohji M, Tano Y. Pars plana vitrectomy with peripheral retinotomy after injection of preoperative intravitreal tissue plasminogen activator: a modified procedure to drain massive subretinal haemorrhage. Br J Ophthalmol [Evaluation Studies Research Support, Non-U.S. Gov't]. 2007;91(2):193–8.
23. Luke M, Januschowski K, Warga M, Beutel J, Leitritz M, Gelisken F, et al. The retinal tolerance to bevacizumab in co-application with a recombinant tissue plasminogen activator. Br J Ophthalmol. 2007;91(8):1077–82.

24. Martin DF, Maguire MG, Fine SL, Ying GS, Jaffe GJ, Grunwald JE, et al. Ranibizumab and bevacizumab for treatment of neovascular age-related macular degeneration: two-year results. Ophthalmology. [Comparative Study Multicenter Study Randomized Controlled Trial Research Support, N.I.H., Extramural]. 2012;119(7):1388–98.
25. Heier JS, Brown DM, Chong V, Korobelnik JF, Kaiser PK, Nguyen QD, et al. Intravitreal aflibercept (VEGF trap-eye) in wet age-related macular degeneration. Ophthalmology. [Clinical Trial, Phase III Comparative Study Multicenter Study Randomized Controlled Trial Research Support, Non-U.S. Gov't]. 2012;119(12):2537–48.
26. van Zeeburg EJ, van Meurs JC. Literature review of recombinant tissue plasminogen activator used for recent-onset submacular hemorrhage displacement in age-related macular degeneration. Ophthalmol J [Research Support, Non-U.S. Gov't Review]. 2013; 229(1):1–14.
27. Kamei M, Misono K, Lewis H. A study of the ability of tissue plasminogen activator to diffuse into the subretinal space after intravitreal injection in rabbits. Am J Ophthalmol. 1999;128(6):739–46.
28. Kwan AS, Vijayasekaran S, McAllister IL, Yu PK, Yu DY. A study of retinal penetration of intravitreal tenecteplase in pigs. Invest Ophthalmol Vis Sci [Research Support, Non-U.S. Gov't]. 2006;47(6): 2662–7.
29. Lincoff H, Madjarov B, Lincoff N, Movshovich A, Saxena S, Coleman DJ, et al. Pathogenesis of the vitreous cloud emanating from subretinal hemorrhage. Arch Ophthalmol [Research Support, Non-U.S. Gov't]. 2003; 121(1):91–6.
30. McAllister IL, Vijayasekaran S, Yu DY. Intravitreal tenecteplase (metalyse) for acute management of retinal vein occlusions. Invest Ophthalmol Vis Sci. [Research Support, Non-U.S. Gov't]. 2013;54(7): 4910–8.

Macular Translocation

8

Gabor B. Scharioth

Introduction

Since its introduction intravitreal anti-VEGF therapy (ranibizumab, bevacizumab) for neovascular age-related macular degeneration has improved the therapeutical options and outcomes for patients with neovascular age-related macular degeneration [1–4].

However, surgical treatment of neovascular AMD in the age of anti-VEGF therapy could be still indicated in patients with nonresponse to intravitreal therapy or large subretinal haemorrhage. Pars plana vitrectomy with subretinal surgery including lavage and removal of choroidal neovascularization was proposed in the late 1990s. But a large prospective study could not show favourable outcome to the natural course [5–8]. In almost all cases, choroidal neovascularization is extending under the fovea, and an extraction will cause a large central retinal pigment epithelium defect. This will result in immediate central scotoma and drop of visual acuity. Furthermore most of large subretinal haemorrhages are caused by rupture of the retinal pigment epithelium. So even after spontaneous resorption of blood or surgical intervention, the visual outcome might be limited due to subfoveal retinal pigment epithelium defect. One solution might be transplantation of an autologous RPE-choroid patch graft to the subfoveal area. But only very limited data are available to support the surgical approach. Furthermore a retrospective review of eyes after full macular translocation (FMT) versus autologous RPE-choroid patch graft in patients with wet AMD found better outcomes in the FMT group, and the authors did recommend FMT in preference to PG. Full macular translocation was first described by Machemer and Steinhorst in 1993 [9, 10]. But FMT was an extremely difficult surgery in these early days of vitreoretinal surgery. There was a lack of sufficient instrumentation and visualization causing relatively high complication rate. Furthermore there was no method developed to treat resulting tilted vision [11]. But later Eckardt, Pertile and others promoted FMT again [12–14]. Microscope-mounted wide-angle viewing systems, endoillumination with chandelier, special instrumentation, shortened surgical time, etc. reduced complication rate and improved outcome. Toth, Neugebauer and others developed modifications of strabismus surgical procedures to address the large-angle cyclotorsion induced by macular translocation surgery for severe age-related macular degeneration [15, 16] (Figs. 8.1, 8.2, 8.3, 8.4, 8.5, 8.6, 8.7, 8.8, 8.9, 8.10, 8.11, 8.12, 8.13, 8.14, 8.15, 8.16, 8.17, 8.18, 8.19, 8.20, 8.21, 8.22 and 8.23).

G.B. Scharioth, M.D., Ph.D.
Aurelios Augenzentrum, Recklinghhausen, Germany

University of Szeged, Szeged, Hungary
e-mail: Gabor.Scharioth@augenzentrum.org

L.-O. Hattenbach (ed.), *Management of Macular Hemorrhage*,
https://doi.org/10.1007/978-3-319-65877-3_8

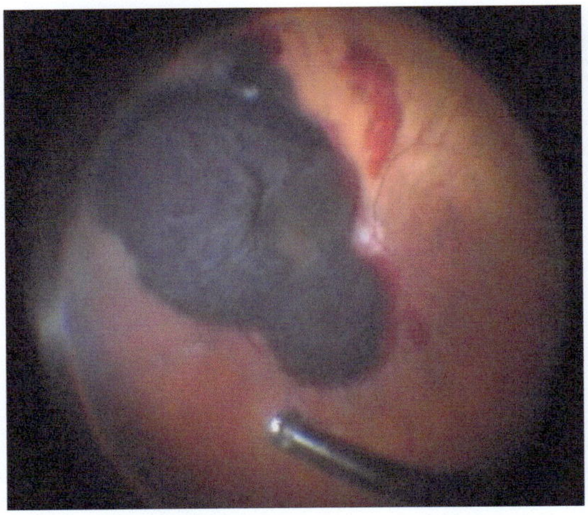

Fig. 8.1 Massive subretinal haemorrhage involving the macula and extending over temporal arcades

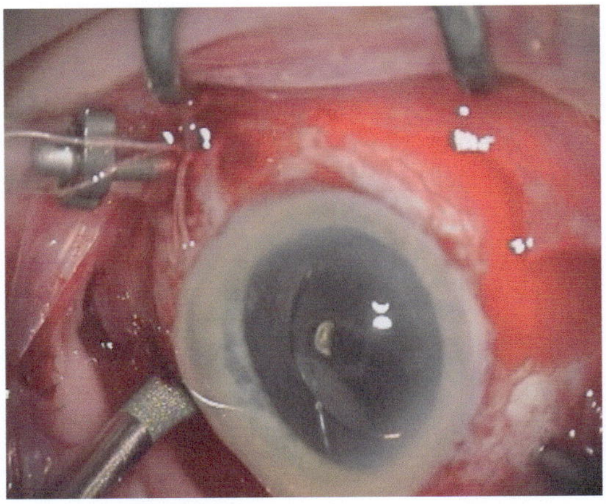

Fig. 8.2 Vitrectomy is completed with vitreous base shaving; a diamond dusted scleral depressor is used for better scleral grip

Surgical Technique

Surgery is performed under general anaesthesia. In selected cases and compliant patient, it might be performed also under retrobulbar anaesthesia. A 360° conjunctival peritomy is performed. If the eye is not already pseudophakic, phacoemulsification through a small incision with implantation

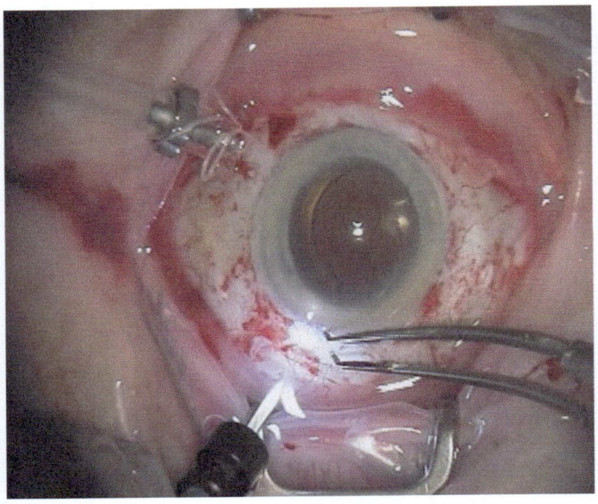

Fig. 8.3 25G chandelier illuminator is placed 3.5 mm postlimbal; alternatively a twin light illuminator could be used to reduce shadowing from instruments

of a foldable acrylic intraocular lens is performed. If needed main incision is secured with a 10 × 0 nylon suture. A three-port 20G pars plana vitrectomy including extensive shaving of the vitreous base is performed. It is mandatory to remove the vitreous completely. Residual vitreous strands might cause intraoperative complications like vitreous-retinal incarceration into the sclerotomies. Next retinal detachment is introduced via three to four microretinotomies with a 41G cannula (DORC, Netherlands) and subretinal balanced salt solution injection (BSS Plus, Alcon, USA). For this a silicone oil injection system is filled with BSS Plus and connected to the vitrectomy machine. Linear foot pedal control improves control of subretinal fluid injection. After multiple large retinal detachment bubbles have formed, it is useful to perform multiple fluid-air exchanges. This further mobilizes the retina. Then the peripheral retina is cut with an endoscissors about 1 mm posterior to the ora serrata circumferentially. We prefer scleral indentation and direct microscope view during this step. But retinotomy could be performed also under visualization with a wide-angle viewing system. Especially

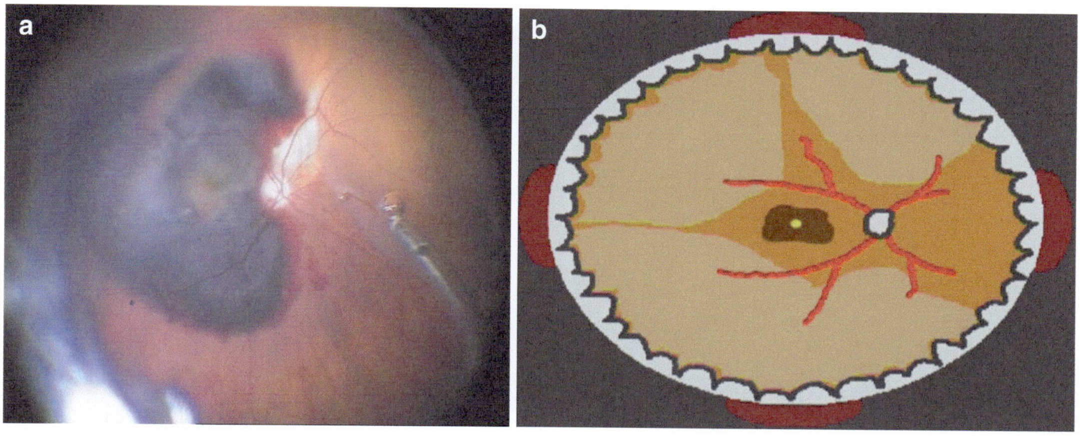

Fig. 8.4 (**a**) Retinal detachment is introduced using a double-bored flute needle with 41G polyamide tip, after creating multiple small retinotomies, and almost complete detachment of multiple fluid-air exchange helps to further mobilize the retina. (**b**) Illustrating situation with detached retina after subretinal fluid injection

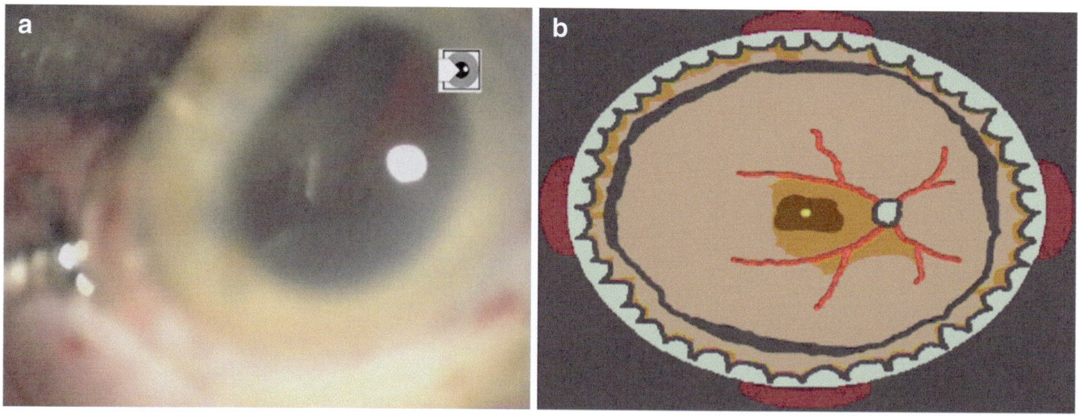

Fig. 8.5 (**a**) Vertical endoscissors is used to create a 360° retinotomy very close to the ora serrata; in eyes with massive subretinal haemorrhage up to periphery recurrent prolapse, blood is often disturbing the view; in such a case peripheral retinotomy is perfomed with a vitreous cutter; the continuous aspiration helps to control the situation. (**b**) Illustrating situation after 360 retinotomy

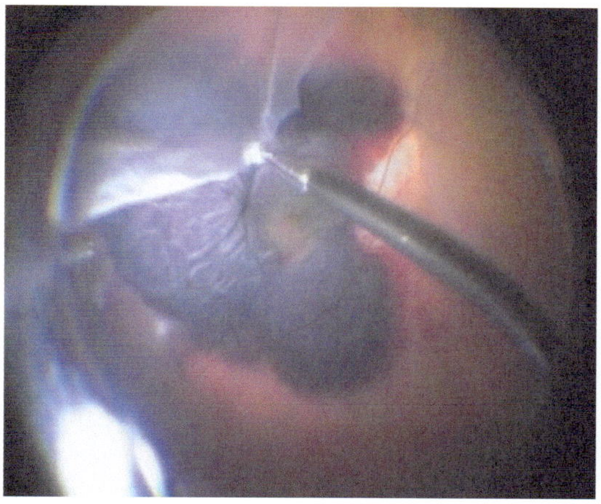

Fig. 8.6 With an atraumatic forceps (e.g. ring forceps) peripheral retina is grasped and mobilized

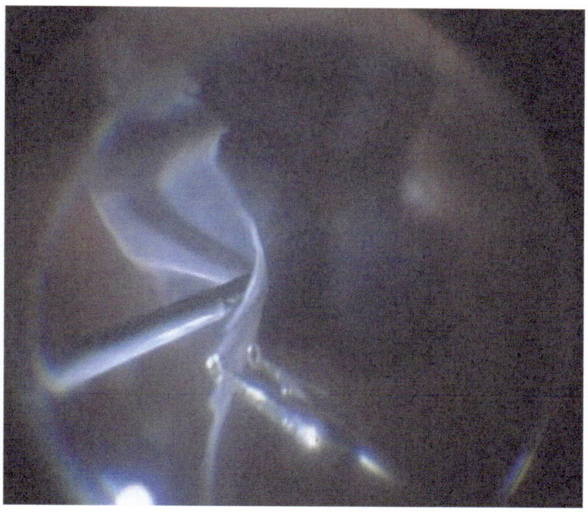

Fig. 8.7 Bimanual manipulation is needed to complete retinal mobilization and to reach subretinal space

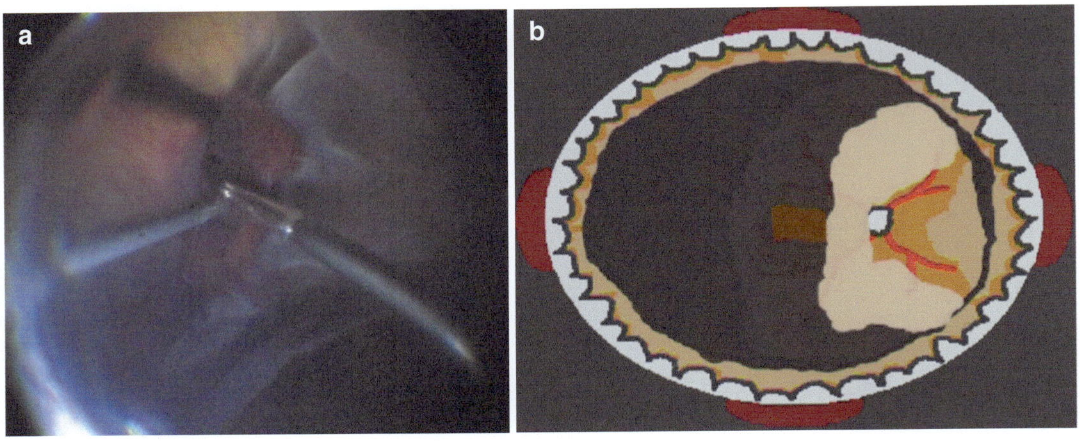

Fig. 8.8 (**a**) Retina is placed to nasal side and stabilized with one forceps; second forceps is used to grasp subretinal coagulum and choroidal neovascular membrane. (**b**) Illustrating situation with retina folded to nasal side to facilitate subretinal manipulations

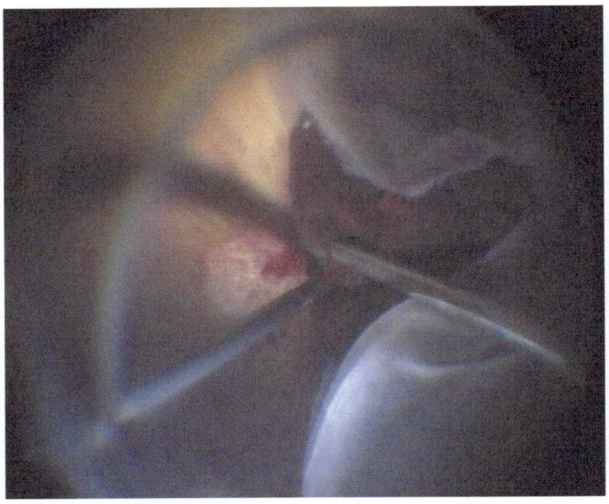

Fig. 8.9 Bimanual manipulation is mandatory; mobilization and separation of choroidal neovascular membrane are often easier if one is able to grasp the nasal edge and pull away from the optic disc; note retinal pigment epithelium defect after CNV is removed

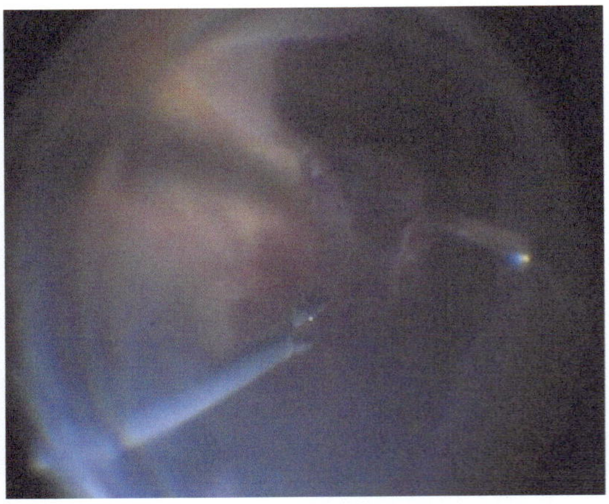

Fig. 8.10 Sometimes it might be useful to change instruments, here the left hand now holds an endgripping forceps

rated forceps. As the optic disc is nasally located from the anatomic axis, the temporal retina is longer. We first grasp the temporal peripheral retina and pull the retina then towards the nasal sclerotomy. This will create a retinal fold. Now we grasp the retinal fold from the subretinal side with the second forceps. This will allow the surgeon to get better access to the submacular region. If retina is not fully mobilized, we pull very carefully to complete detachment. Sometimes it might be useful to use the second instrument as a counter pole to pull around. During this step again, prolapsing blood might diminish the view. Lavage with vitrectome or Charles needle might be necessary. To prevent aspiration of the mobile retina, we hold the retina with the Endo Forceps. Subretinal blood and the subfoveal choroidal neovascularization are removed. In our experience it might be easier to grasp the subretinal complex from the papillary side and pull the coagulum-choroidal neovascular membrane complex towards the peripheral retina. All these steps are truly bimanual manipulations. Sometimes this complex is so large that it

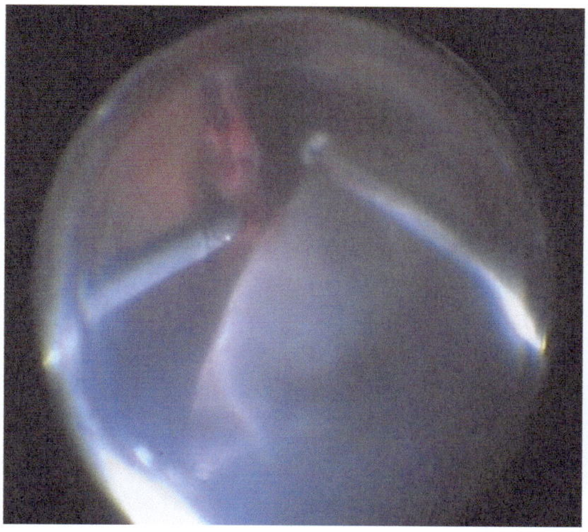

Fig. 8.11 Left forceps is holding the nasal edge of choroidal neovascular complex, prolapsing blood was aspirated with vitreous cutter in the right hand, and in case of extremely large subretinal blood coagulum, sometimes the cutter is used to reduce its size

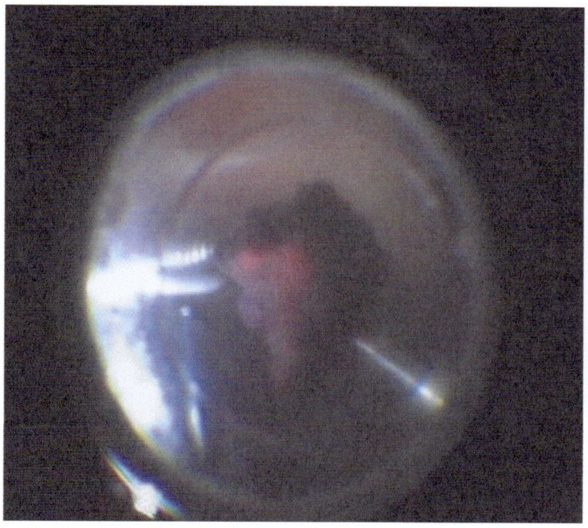

Fig. 8.12 Choroidal neovascular membrane and coagulum is prolapse from subretinal space into the vitreous cavity and lifted behind the intraocular lens; now it can be cut and aspirated in the safe zone

in case of blood reflux from subretinal space, the fundus view might be diminished. In this situation the surgeon might use a vitrectome to perform the retinotomy. The simultaneous aspiration and cutting reduce blood reflux into the vitreous cavity. A chandelier illuminator is placed at 12 o'clock position 3.5 mm posterior to the limbus, and the retina is mobilized bimanually to get access to the subretinal space. We prefer in one hand a ring forceps and in the other hand a ser-

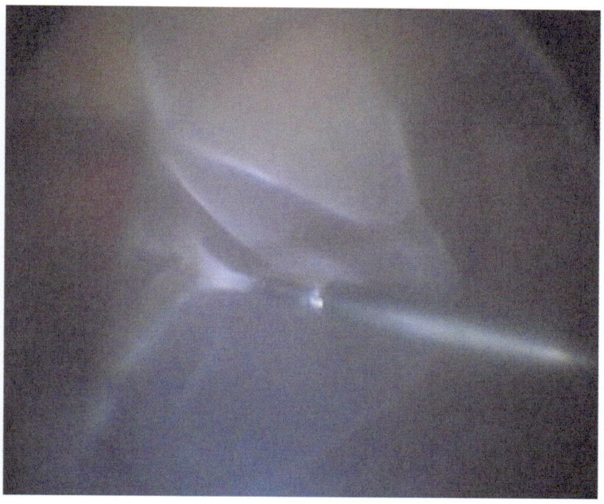

Fig. 8.13 Right hand holds retina with an atraumatic forceps (e.g. ring forceps or silcone tipped forceps) from outer side and pulls carefully towards nasal side, note retinal folds

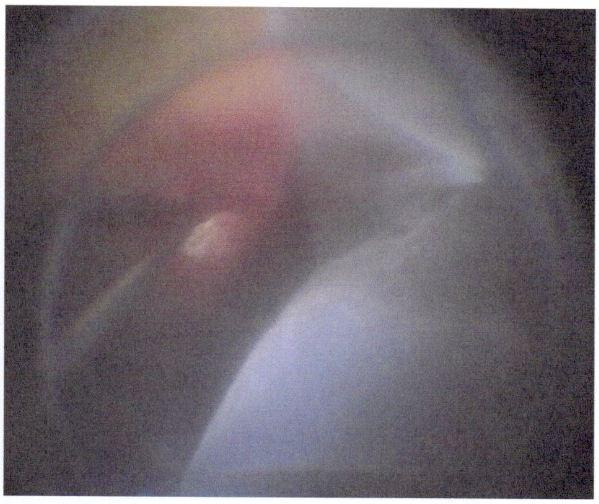

Fig. 8.14 Charles flute needle is used with passive aspiration to remove bleeding from the submacular area

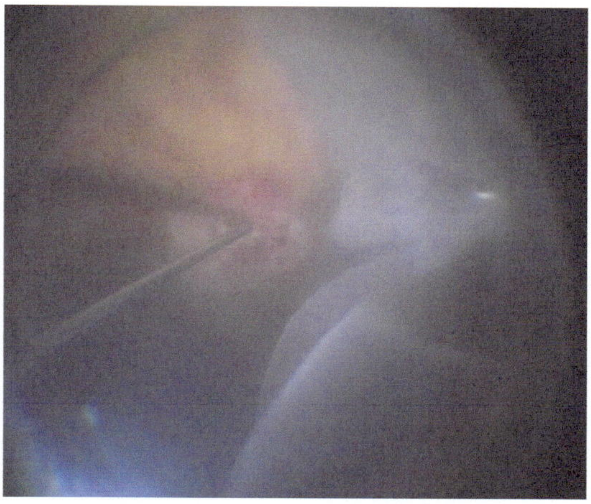

Fig. 8.15 Endodiathermy is used to stop bleeding from feeder vessel

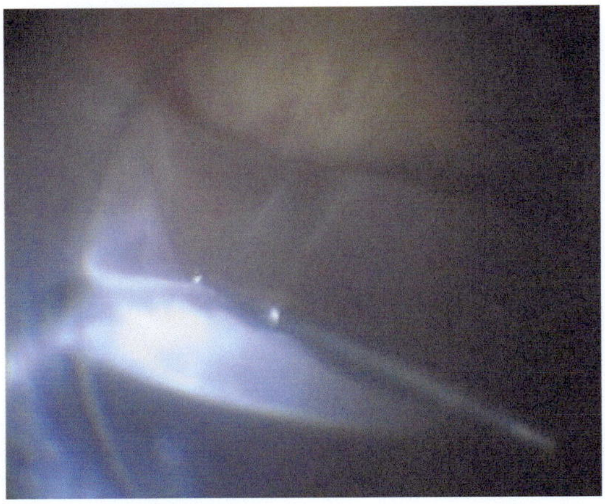

Fig. 8.16 Retinal detachment is completed, one forceps holds retinal edge, while second forceps is used to mobilize the retina; it is important that retinal detachment is completed till optic disc

cannot be removed through the sclerotomy. In such case we use the vitrectome with reduced cutting rate to remove the coagulum. The complex is held in the safe zone behind the intraocular lens to prevent unwanted retinal aspiration. In some rare cases, the residual CNV is so large and dense that it cannot be removed through the sclerotomies or via vitrectome. In this situation a second Endo Forceps is used, and the CNV is torn into smaller pieces. Typically the removal of CNV results in a submacular defect of the retinal pigment epithelium. If the feeder vessel bleeds or diffuse bleeding comes from the CNV bed, endodiathermy might be needed. We prefer a pointed 25 G endodiathermy probe to minimize collateral damage. Retina is then refolded and stabilized with a bubble of heavy fluid (F6H8, Geuder,

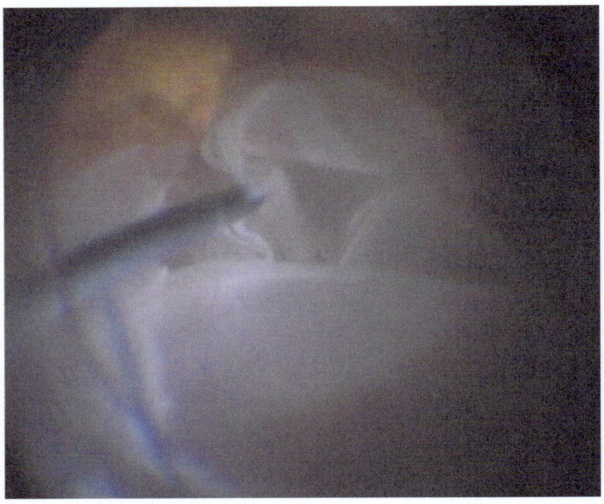

Fig. 8.17 Retinal edge is grasped with forceps before heavy liquid is injected

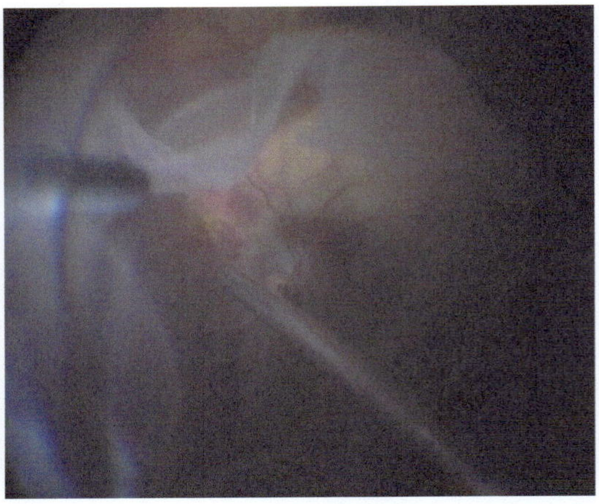

Fig. 8.18 Using a double-bored flute needle slowly, heavy liquid is injected to unfold and reattach the retina

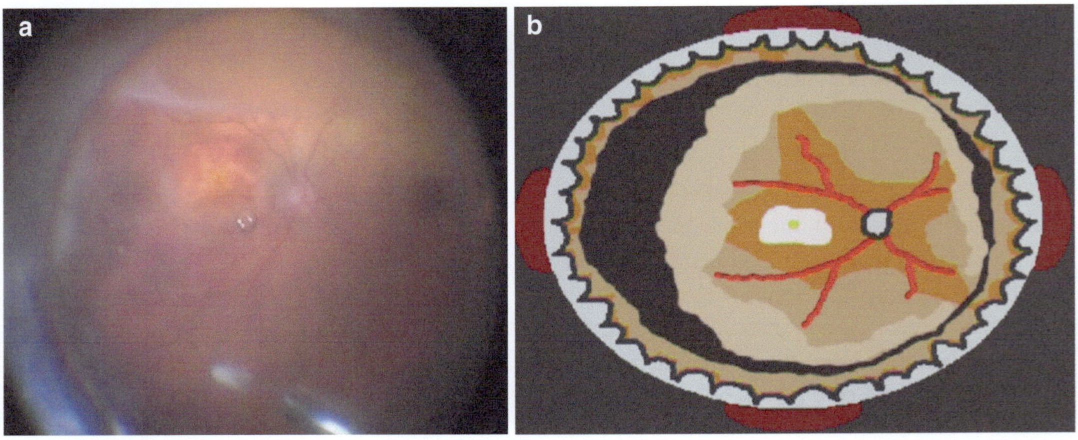

Fig. 8.19 Heavy fluid is injected until the retina is attached up to midperiphery; note that fovea is placed over the retinal pigment epithelium defect. (**a**) Illustrating situation with partially reattached retina under PFCL

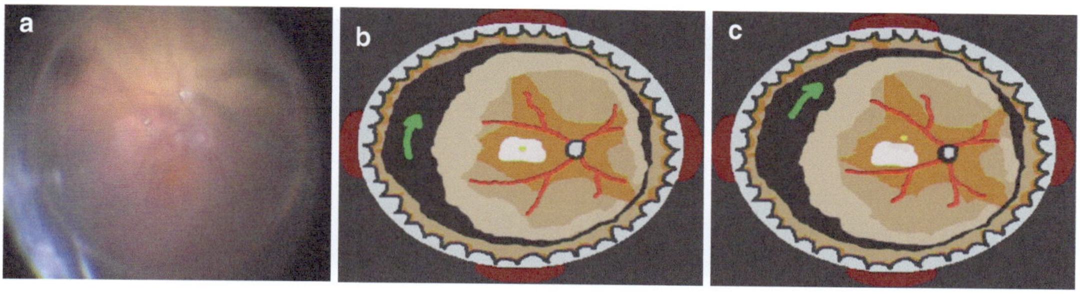

Fig. 8.20 (**a**) Diamond duster sweeper or a silicone-tipped flute needle is used to rotate the retina; note that fovea is placed upwards outside the retinal pigment epithelium defect. (**b**) Illustrating situation before macular translocation, note that this is not an intraoperative surgeon's view; it shows the situation in a sitting position. (**c**) Illustrating situation after upward rotation of the retina, fovea is placed away from the retinal pigment epithelium defect; note that this is not an intraoperative surgeon's view; it shows situation in a sitting position

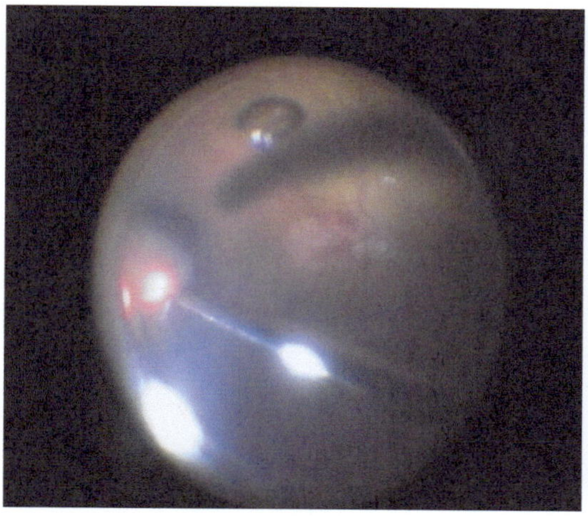

Fig. 8.21 Peripheral circumferential laser retinopexy is performed; for better visualization scleral indentation is used; overlapping retina in superior and nasal-superior periphery is trimmed with vitreous cutter

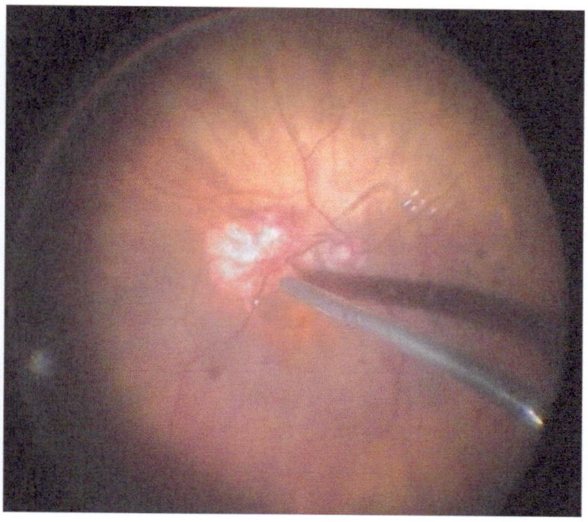

Fig. 8.22 Direct heavy fluid—silicone oil—exchange is performed; while silicone oil is injected under linear control of the machine, the heavy fluid is passively aspirated through a flute needle, to prevent excessive intraocular pressure rise; the last bubble of heavy fluid is aspirated actively (e.g. introducing the flute needle into the heavy fluid bubble with compressed silicone reservoir; release of the reservoir creates enough vacuum to aspirate the remaining small bubble

Germany). We prefer F6H8 because it is less heavy than Decalin, and by this retinal receptor damage might be reduced during translocation. The retina is flattened up to midperiphery. Macular translocation around the optic nerve head in the upward direction is performed with the help of an atraumatic diamond dusted sweeper (DORC, Netherlands) or a silicone-tipped aspiration needle. If possible we prefer upward-directed rotation. As the retinal pigment epithelium defect will result in a scotoma around the temporal arcade, we believe that a superior scotoma is less irritating to the patient. An inferior scotoma will not just irritate during reading but also during walking, stepping, etc. The retina is only rotated downwards if the extent of the retinal pigment epithelium defect does not allow foveal placement onto unaffected retinal pigment epithelium. But inferior macular translocation also would increase the risk of macular involvement in case of postoperative inferior retinal detachment. Next the retina is completely attached by further injection of heavy fluid (Decalin, Geuder, Germany) up to the pars plana. Under light scleral indentation, peripheral laser retinopexy is applied circumferentially, and the overlapping retinal edge in the upper half is trimmed. Finally a direct heavy fluid—silicone oil—exchange is performed. We prefer silicone oil injection via infusion line and passive Decalin aspiration via

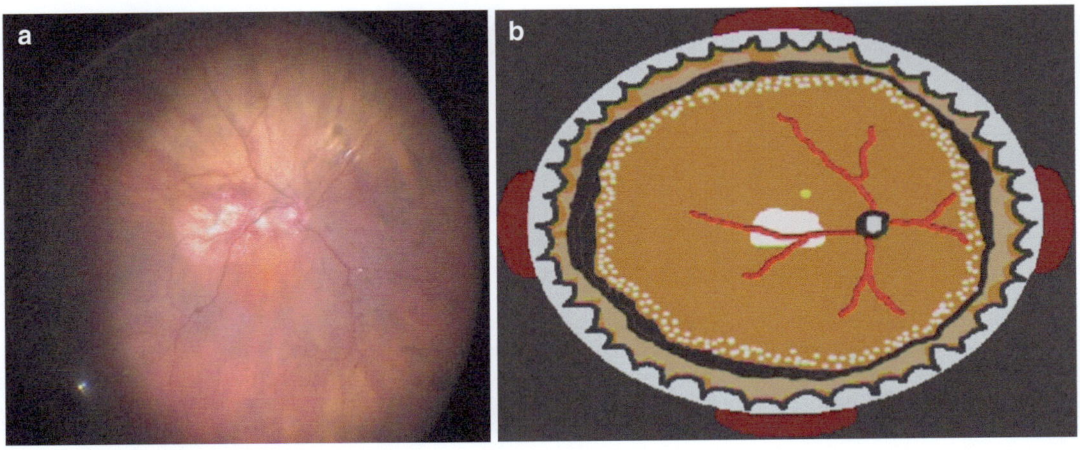

Fig. 8.23 (**a**) Final situation after full macular translocation, complete silicone oil fill, retina upwards rotated, macula outside the retinal pigment epithelium defect. (**b**) Illustrating final situation with upward rotated retina, fovea placed outside the retinal pigment epithelium defect, circumferential peripheral laser retinopexy and silicone oil tamponade, note that this s not an intraoperative surgeon's view; it shows situation in a sitting position

Charles aspiration cannula. To prevent extremely high intraocular pressure, the last Decalin bubbles are actively aspirated. A "Staubsauger" with a large silicone reservoir is used. The reservoir is pressed and just released if the needle enters the remaining Decalin bubble. In case of subretinal Decalin, a microretinotomy is created and Decalin is aspirated. Intraocular pressure is checked. Sclerotomies and conjunctiva are closed with adsorbable sutures (Vicryl 8/0, Ethicon) (Figs. 8.24, 8.25 and 8.26).

Postoperative therapy includes hourly cortisone eye drops (e.g. prednisolone 1%, URSAPHARM, Germany) and antibiotic ointment four times daily. During the first postoperative days, the patient is asked to change every 4 h position from left to right side. This will move the intraocular silicone oil bubble and help to keep the inferior retina attached. We found a dramatic drop of inferior retinal detachment rate after starting this postoperative positioning regimen.

Three months after initial surgery, counterrotation with transposition of the horizontal and oblique muscles in combination with pars plana vitrectomy and silicone oil removal is performed. Some surgeons advocate for surgery of oblique muscles only, whereas others prefer to split all straight muscles and transposition a part under the neighbouring muscle on its other side.

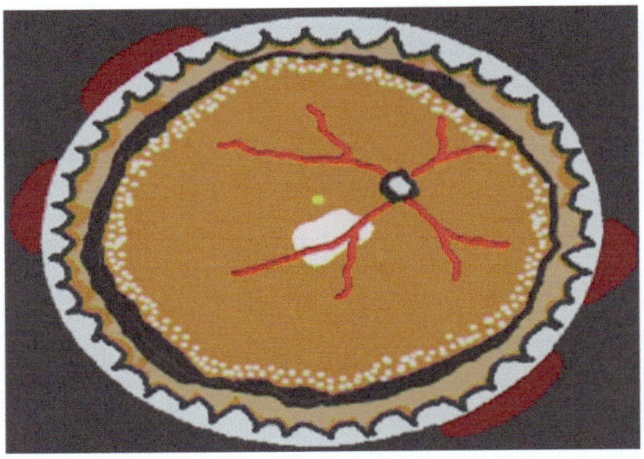

Fig. 8.24 Illustrating situation after counterrotation and repositioning of external muscles

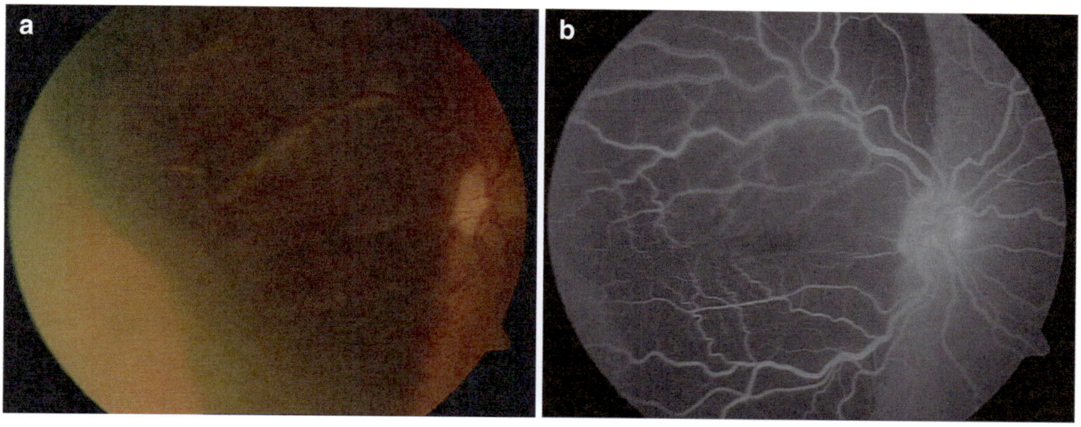

Fig. 8.25 (**a**) Fundus photo of a single-eyed 82-year-old male with massive subretinal haemorrhage, sudden visual loss few days before, visual acuity only hand motion. (**b**) Fluorescence angiography of same eye

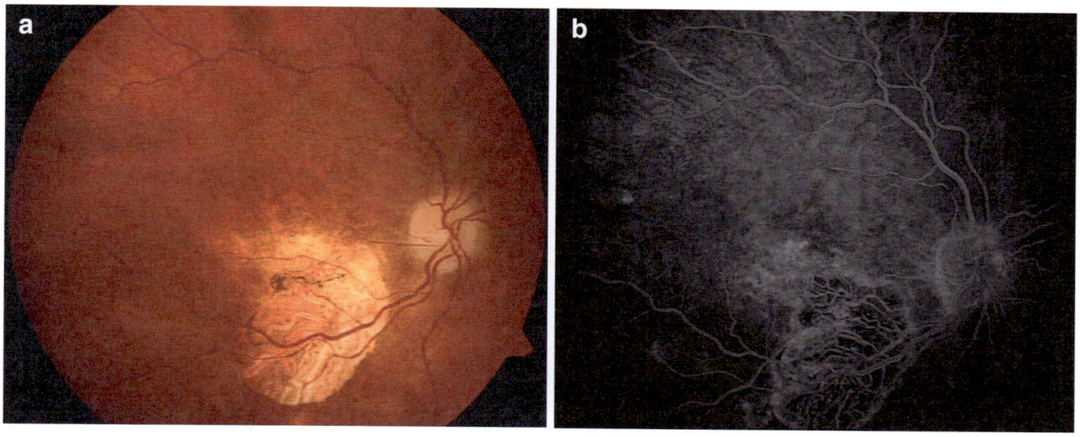

Fig. 8.26 (**a**) Fundus photo of the same eye 3 years after pars plana vitrectomy with full macular translocation, visual acuity improved to 0.25, patient is able to read the newspaper with the help of low vision aids. (**b**) Fluorescence angiography of the same eye 3 years after pars plana vitrectomy with full macular translocation; note: no sign of CNV recurrence or cystoid macular oedema

References

1. Martin DF, Maguire MG, Fine SL, et al. Ranibizumab and bevacizumab for treatment of neovascular age-related macular degeneration: two-year results. Ophthalmology. 2012;119(7):1388–98.
2. Congdon N, O'Colmain B, Klaver CC, et al. Causes and prevalence of visual impairment among adults in the United States. Arch Ophthalmol. 2004;122(4):477–85.
3. Rosenfeld PJ, Brown DM, Heier JS, et al. Ranibizumab for neovascular age-related macular degeneration. N Engl J Med. 2006;355(14):1419–31.
4. Heier JS, Brown DM, Chong V, et al. Intravitreal aflibercept (VEGF trap-eye) in wet age-related macular degeneration. Ophthalmology. 2012;119(12):2537–48.
5. Submacular Surgery Trials (SST) Research Group. Surgery for subfoveal choroidal neovascularization in age-related macular degeneration: ophthalmic findings. SST report no. 11. Ophthalmology. 2004;111:1967–80.
6. Submacular Surgery Trials (SST) Research Group. Surgery for subfoveal choroidal neovascularization in age-related macular degeneration: quality-of-life findings. SST report no. 12. Ophthalmology. 2004;111:1981–92.

7. Submacular Surgery Trials (SST) Research Group. Surgery for hemorrhagic choroidal neovascular lesions of age-related macular degeneration: ophthalmic findings. SST report no. 13. Ophthalmology. 2004;111:1993–2006.
8. Submacular Surgery Trials (SST) Research Group. Surgery for hemorrhagic choroidal neovascular lesions of age-related macular degeneration: quality-of-life findings. SST report no 14. Ophthalmology. 2004;111:2007–14.
9. Machemer R, Steinhorst UH. Retinal separation, retinotomy, and macular relocation: I. Experimental studies in rabbit eye. Graefes Arch Clin Exp Ophthalmol. 1993;231:629–34.
10. Machemer R, Steinhorst UH. Retinal separation, retinotomy, and macular relocation: II. A surgical approach for age-related macular degeneration? Graefes Arch Clin Exp Ophthalmol. 1993;231: 635–41.
11. Eckardt U, Eckardt C. [Orthoptic problems after macular rotation with and without muscle surgery]. Klin Monbl Augenheilkd. 1998;212(4):212–7. German.
12. Eckardt C, Eckardt U, Conrad HG. Macular rotation with and without counter-rotation of the globe in patients with age-related macular degeneration. Graefes Arch Clin Exp Ophthalmol. 1999 Apr;237(4):313–25.
13. Au Eong KG, Pieramici DJ, Fujii GY, Ng EW, Humayun MS, Maia M, Harlan JB Jr, Schachat AP, Beatty S, Toth CA, Thomas MA, Lewis H, Eckardt C, Tano Y, de Juan E. Macular translocation: unifying concepts, terminology, and classification. Am J Ophthalmol. 2001;131(2):244–53, Review.
14. Pertile G, Claes C. Macular translocation with 360 degree retinotomy for management of age-related macular degeneration with subfoveal choroidal neovascularization. Am J Ophthalmol. 2002;134(4):560–5.
15. Freedman SF, Rojas M, Toth CA. Strabismus surgery for large-angle cyclotorsion after macular translocation surgery. J AAPOS. 2002;6(3):154–62. Erratum in: J AAPOS 2002;6(4):246.
16. Fricke J, Neugebauer A, Nobis H, et al. Counterrotation of the globe in macular translocation. Graefes Arch Clin Exp Ophthalmol. 2000;238:664–8.

Autologous Choroidal RPE Patch Transplantation in Hemorrhagic Age-Related Macular Degeneration

9

Barbara Parolini, Attilio Di Salvatore, and Alessandro Finzi

Introduction

Various types of exudative maculopathies have in common a primary damage to the retinal pigment epithelium (RPE) and a secondary damage of the retina. Autologous transplantation of RPE and choroid (RPE-choroidal patch) is a surgical technique that has the rationale to transport healthy RPE and choroid, from the periphery to the location under the macula, when the original RPE is damaged by atrophic changes or by choroidal subfoveal neovascularization.

This method was first described by Peyman and associates in 1991 [1]. Aylward [2] introduced the concept of a free patch in six patients, taken from an area directly adjacent to the excised choroidal membrane. Van Meurs modified the technique by harvesting the patch from the midperiphery [3].

In previous years, a transplantation of a suspension of autologous RPE cells, harvested from the periphery during submacular surgery for removal of the hemorrhage/CNV, had been proposed, but this surgery has shown limited benefits [4]. In fact, cell suspensions have difficulties attaching to the diseased Bruch's membrane and often do not form the desired monolayer required for optimal RPE function and undergo a form of apoptosis. An RPE-choroidal patch may provide a better cell sourcew with more chance of regaining normal retinal structures and thus visual acuity [5].

Van Zeeburg et al. suggested that RPE-choroidal patch may be an alternative for patients with AMD who have not benefitted from, or cannot undergo, other standard treatments [6, 7], but they also show that a higher gain in vision might be possible for patients with a RPE-choroidal patch instead of anti-VEGF treatment, in the absence of complications [8].

Autologous Transplantation of RPE and Choroid: Surgical Technique

In 2011, we reported on the feasibility and safety of the RPE-choroidal patch with a different surgical technique, through a peripheral retinotomy, in order to lower the chance of complications [9]. A 20 ga pars plana vitrectomy is extended to the vitreous base and verified multiple times with triamcinolone. The inferotemporal sclerotomy is cut perpendicularly and occupied by an illuminated infusion cannula, sutured to the sclera. The superior sclerotomies are cut tangentially to the scleral plane. Residues of vitreous should be aspirated and removed with the vitrectomy probe. After peeling of the internal limiting membrane (ILM), a retinal detachment is induced by injecting balanced salt solution into the subretinal space through a 41g needle, connected to an

B. Parolini, M.D. (✉) · A. Di Salvatore, M.D.
A. Finzi, M.D.
Istituto Clinico S.Anna, Brescia, Italy

L.-O. Hattenbach (ed.), *Management of Macular Hemorrhage*,
https://doi.org/10.1007/978-3-319-65877-3_9

active pump of the vitrectomy machine. The retinal detachment is completed with a fluid air exchange. Under fluid, a roughly 200° peripheral retinotomy is performed with scissors at the ora serrata, from 10–11 o'clock to 5–6 o'clock. The temporal retina is then folded on the nasal retina to discover the temporal superior and inferior subretinal space. CNVs are removed with forceps and spatula. Subretinal blood is aspirated with the vitrectomy probe. Endodiathermy is applied to the feeder vessels after CNV removal. Endodiathermy is also applied in other spots of the submacular choroid, with the aim to create a microtrauma into the choriocapillaris and favor the revascularization of the patch. The location of the harvesting site of the patch is chosen by visually selecting an area of normally appearing RPE and trying to avoid the vortex veins. The area is mainly chosen in the temporal quadrant, superiorly or inferiorly, and traced with confluent endolaser spots or with endodiathermy, directed on the RPE. A full thickness patch of RPE and choroid is isolated with scissors and, simultaneously, choroidal bleeding controlled by endodiathermy and aspiration of the blood. After cutting the posterior half perimeter of the patch, perfluorocarbon liquid (PFCL) is injected into the subretinal space and onto the isolated edges of the patch, in order to avoid the rolling and elevation of the edges of the patch. Then, the second anterior half of the patch is cut and transplanted with a non-toothed forceps, in the area corresponding to the macula, under PFCL. Care should be taken to flatten the border of the patch with a spatula.

In the harvesting site, the residues of choroid are removed from the sclera with aspiration and\ or forceps. The borders of the choroid, in the harvesting site, are intensively treated with endodiathermy. PFCL is progressively and slowly aspirated and reinjected in the epiretinal space in order to flatten the retina on top of the patch and to center the fovea on visually healthy RPE. If the patch is not centered, PFCL is moved again subretinally, the patch is centered, and then the maneuver of shifting PFCL from the subretinal to the epiretinal space is repeated. The retina is then completely reattached with PFCL and the retinotomy sealed with multiple rows of laser, followed by a peripheral 360° endolaser cerclage. The peripheral retina at the ora serrata anterior to the retinotomy is carefully removed using the vitrectomy probe. PFCL is then exchanged directly with silicone oil 1000. Silicone oil should be removed after at least 3 months.

Clinical Outcome

The long-term functional results and the complication rate of our modified RPE-choroidal patch technique were investigated in a series of eyes with hemorrhagic age-related macular degeneration (Hem-AMD). The functional results are reported not only in terms of visual acuity but also, for a subgroup of patients, with a Macular Integrity Assessment Device (MAIA) system to test the retina sensitivity and locus of fixation. MAIA provides accurate and objective information regarding retinal location and stability of a patient's fixation. Such parameters are assessed by tracking eye movements 25 times/s and by plotting the resulting distribution over the SLO image. Each movement is represented by a point in the distribution. We also used low vision test, consisting of 68 test loci covering the central 20°, with a 4-2 projection strategy, which changes the light intensity in 4 dB steps until there is a change from not seen to seen (or from seen to not seen). Then the intensity changes in 2 db steps until the stimulus is not seen again. Secondary outcomes included the description of the patch evolution at biomicroscopy, optical coherence tomography (OCT), fluorescein angiography (FA), indocyanine green (ICG), and autofluorescence (AF).

Inclusion criteria were CNV secondary to AMD in patients with RPE tear and subretinal hemorrhages or patients losing vision after at least the sixth anti-VEGF injection. Of a cohort of 120 patients with atrophic or exudative maculopathies who received RPE patch surgery, complete data for analysis were collected for 23 patients with a diagnosis of hemorrhagic retinal detachment due to choroidal neovascularization (CNV) and age-related macular degeneration (AMD). The follow-up was at least 24 months. Reading ability was defined as ability to read at least point 12 of print letters.

Functional Results

The mean preoperative BCVA was 1.2 logMar and the mean final BCVA was 1 logMar. The difference was statistically significant with a p value <0.05. (Table 9.1) reports the number and percentage of eyes presenting with preoperative and final BCVA $\leq$1 logMar, BCVA $\leq$0.5 logMar, and BCVA $\leq$0.3 logMar. The mean time to recover the final vision was 12 months.

(Table 9.2) shows the letters lost and gained as well as the gained reading ability after surgery.

Considering the functional situation of the fellow eye, seven fellow eyes (30%) had BCVA >1 logMar. In the group of patients with BCVA >1 logMar in the fellow eye, the average final vision in the operated eye was 1.1 logMar.

Microperimetry

A subgroup of three eyes, with final reading ability of at least 12pt, underwent microperimetry, which became available only recently. All eyes showed a central foveal fixation with average sensitivity of 10.5 dB (range 5.1–14.8 dB) and average fixation stability of $P1 = 37.8\%$ (range 10–87%) and $P2 = 73.5\%$. Fixation was located over the patch.

Complications

The postoperative complications, observed between 10 days and 3 months after surgery, are listed in (Table 9.3). Three eyes with postoperative retinal detachment and four with epiretinal membrane received further surgery, obtaining improvement in vision. The most threatening complication was postoperative subretinal hemorrhage. All the patients who presented this complication were undertaking anticoagulant drugs which had been suspended 15 days prior to surgery. These eyes lost significant vision due to the complications with average final vision of 1.5 logMar.

Surgical Time

The mean surgical time was 2.50 h (range 2.30–4.10) in the first seven eyes and decreased to 1.40 h (range 1.20–2.55) in the subsequent cases.

Anatomical Results

In patients that did not have hazy media, the RPE-choroidal patch was well visible, between 1 day and 1 week post-op, in the subfoveal area as a pigmented thick oval or roundish tissue, with an average size of 3 disc diameters. In the temporal quadrants, a whitish area of bare sclera was visible, identifying the harvesting site of the patch. Subretinal blood remnants at the borders of the harvesting site were a common finding and lasted for the first 4–6 weeks.

One month after surgery, the RPE-choroidal patch had more defined and flat thin edges. A progressive reabsorption of blood was observed at the harvesting site.

Table 9.1 N and percentage of eyes with final BCVA <1 logMar, ≤ 0.5 logMar and ≤ 0.3 logMar

	Preop BCVA ≤ 1 logMar	Final BCVA ≤ 1 logMar	Preop BCVA ≤ 0.5 logMar	Final BCVA ≤ 0.5 logMar	Preop BCVA ≤ 0.3 logMar	Final BCVA ≤ 0.3 logMar
CNV-AMD-H (23 eyes)	3 (13.1%)	11 (47.8%)	0	5 (21.7%)	0	2 (9%)

Table 9.2 Gain in letter score

	Gain of at least 15 letters	Loss of at least 15 letters	Stable (± 5 letters)	Reading ability at the final visit
CNV-AMD-Hem (23 eyes)	11 (47.8%)	1 (4.3%)	8 (34.7%)	10 (43.5%)

Table 9.3 Postoperative complications

Postoperative complications	Rate
Retinal detachment	3 (13%)
Subretinal haemorrhage	2 (4.3%)
Macular hole	1 (4.3%)
Epiretinal membrane	4 (17.4%)
Recurrent CNV	1 (4.3%)
Macular atrophy and cystoid edema	4 (17.4%)

Commonly, the patch had a darker pigmentation with respect to the surrounding tissue.

Silicone oil was removed in 20 patients between 3 and 8 months after surgery. After silicone oil removal, the appearance of the patch and the harvesting site did not change through follow-up. In a subgroup of patients, we could observe a fibrotic thin scar like a whitish prophyle surrounding the patch. The fibrotic scar extended to the harvesting site, in the eyes in which the shortest distance between the edge of the patch and the harvesting site was inferior to the diameter of the harvesting site.

On OCT, the patch was well visible as a subfoveal layer of RPE and choroid with open large hyporeflective spaces corresponding to perfused choroidal vessels. We could observe the disappearance of cystoid macular edema in the early postoperative time when present preoperatively. The visibility of the external layers of the retina changed in time, being barely visible for at least 1 month after surgery and becoming more defined in the following weeks.

Revascularization was observed in 100% of the eyes. One month after surgery, FA and ICG confirmed the vascularization of the patch. The choroidal vessels into the patch presented different direction from the vessels of the surrounding choroid. Some eyes presented a nonhomogeneous vascularization, meaning that some areas of the patch were less vascularized than others and presented sectorial hypoperfusion.

Autofluorescence (AF) was normal over the area of the patch and comparable to the AF of the surrounding choroid. Multiple areas of hypoautofluorescence were noticed at the borders of the patch where the necessary surgical manipulation was applied. Some eyes presented scattered areas of hypoautofluorescence also over the patch more than 6 months.

Complications

We have observed a lower rate of complications compared to what was reported in literature for the same subject. We think that the lower rate of PVR, epiretinal membrane, and macular hole could be related to the different surgical technique implying a peripheral retinotomy and the peeling of the internal limiting membrane. Peripheral laser was applied over the border of the retinotomy and extended 360° only in the presence of rhegmatogenous lesions. Silicone oil 1000 was the only tamponade used.

The lower rate of CNV relapse compared to other reports [7, 10] could be related to the heavy diathermy applied to the feeder vessel after removing the CNV. One more hypothesis is that the patch of peripheral choroid, which is located on top of the macular choroid, increases the local choroidal flow and this prevents new ischemic insult and consequent CNV.

The successful rate of revascularization could be due to the heavy diathermy applied to the macular choroidal surface in multiple areas before transplanting the patch of choroid. We think that this maneuver might create a microtrauma to the choriocapillaris that might favor the revascularization.

Epiretinal membrane could be prevented by applying to all eyes the internal limiting membrane peeling (ILM) at the time of patch surgery, and this was observed by analyzing the lower rate of epiretinal membrane in the eyes operated more recently with the addition of ILM peeling.

The most sight-threatening complication was the postoperative macular atrophy, which was probably due to excessive preoperative external retinal atrophy. Other sight-threatening complications were macular holes and subretinal hemorrhages. Macular holes occurred intraoperatively during the detachment of the retina with subretinal injection. The authors think that to avoid this complication it is recommendable to start detaching the retina, injecting first in the periphery and not in the submacular area. Furthermore, the peeling of internal limiting membrane should be made but foveal sparing in order to avoid weakening the foveal roof during the retinal detachment.

Subretinal hemorrhages occurred in patients who were undertaking anticoagulant therapy. This condition is now considered by the surgeon a strict exclusion criterion.

Conclusions

The transplantation of a full thickness patch of RPE and choroid under the fovea has the potential to improve vision significantly in a selected group of patients affected by hemorrhagic CNV secondary to AMD. In our series, roughly 47.8% of the eyes showed an improvement in vision of at least 15 letters; 34.7% remained stable. This means that 82.5% of these eyes did not experience visual loss in a follow-up as long as 8 years. The mean final vision was significantly improved when compared to the mean preoperative vision. Patients who presented visual improvement not only gained far sight but also reading ability and central fixation. In fact, 43.5% of the patients reached the ability to read again, and do so using the area of retina over the patch, as demonstrated by microperimetry.

BCVA improvement is not immediate. These results resemble the ones obtained by the same surgeon in a larger series of 120 eyes operated for CNV not associated to subretinal hemorrhages, CNV of other etiologies than AMD and for atrophic maculopathies (unpublished data). The follow-up in the present study was at least 2 years. However, ten eyes have a follow-up between 4 and 8 years. The long follow-up has allowed us to understand that eyes that show an improvement in vision do so only after at least 1 year and then show a slow but constant improvement in the following years until reaching the final result roughly 3 years after surgery (unpublished data collected by the surgeon), as previously reported by Van Zeeburg et al. [7, 11]. None of the eyes, which showed an improvement in vision, presented a vision loss after reaching the highest improvement in vision. Patients achieved a gain in vision of at least 15 letters in 47.8% of the eyes.

However, the surgical technique presented here requires a long training and specific instrumentation. Only expert vitreoretinal surgeons can perform this technique. In fact, the operating time decreased to almost half in the last eyes, as well as the occurrence of complications. The authors believe that a significant part of the success of the surgery relies on the intraoperative course, both in terms of efficacy and safety. Two operations are required with the present technique because the tamponade in the first surgery was always silicone oil 1000. The transplant is autologous and therefore the tissue has the same age as the patient.

We think it is important to consider the vision in the fellow eye as well. In many cases, the patients are affected by a bilateral disease. The average BCVA of the fellow eye of the whole group was 0.74 logMar. Seven fellow eyes (30%) had BCVA >1 logMar at the time of surgery, and in this group of patients the final vision in the operated eye was higher than the fellow eye. This element should be considered in the decision-making process that leads to surgery.

Acknowledgments The author has no financial interest in the subject of the paper. I acknowledge Dr. Marco Morales for his insights on the use of MAIA microperimeter.

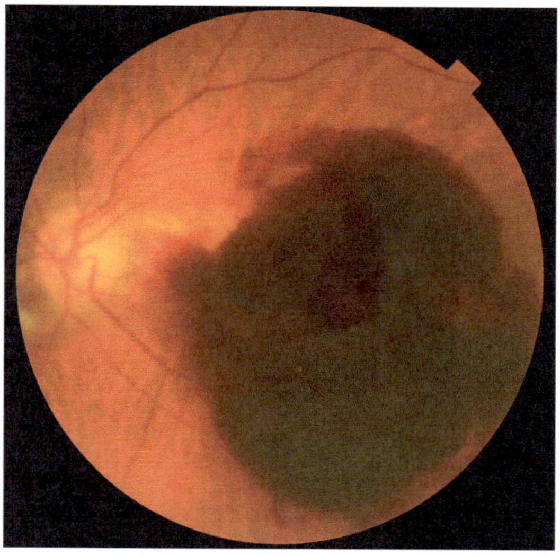

Fig. 9.1 Hemorrhagic retinal detachment of the posterior pole, secondary to age related macular degeneration (AMD) and choroidal neovascularization (CNV)

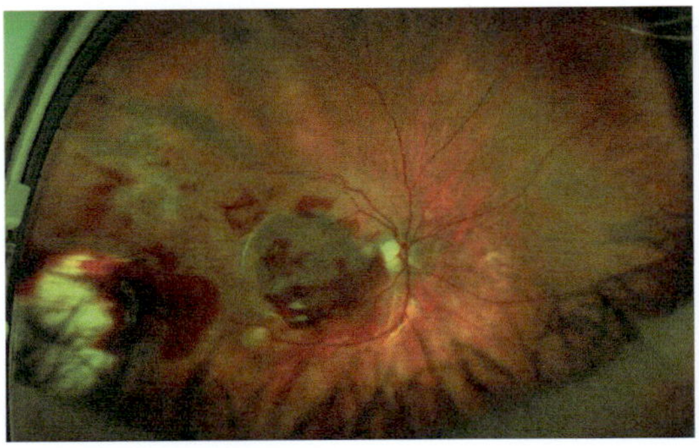

Fig. 9.2 Color fundus picture of postop day 5. A roundish patch of choroid and RPE is visible under the posterior pole. Residues of subretinal blood are present under the posterior pole and the harvesting site in the temporal side

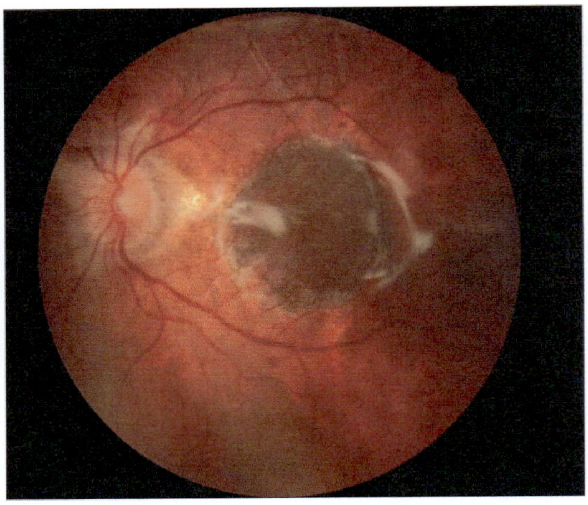

Fig. 9.3 Color fundus picture 1 month postop. A roundish patch of choroid and RPE is visible under the posterior pole. The color of the patch is darker and more brown that the surrounding tissue

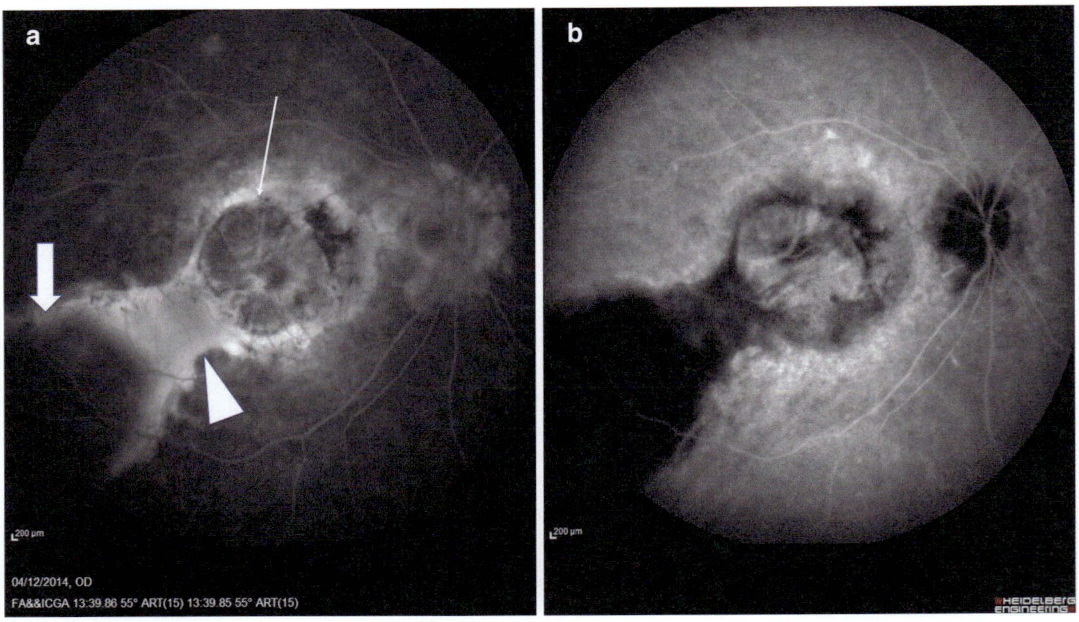

Fig. 9.4 Fluorescein angiography (**a**) and Indocianine green (**b**), 1 month postop. A roundish patch of choroid and RPE is visible under the posterior pole. The patch (arrow line) is surrounded by a fibrotic scar (arrowhead) that extends to the harvesting site (thick white arrow)

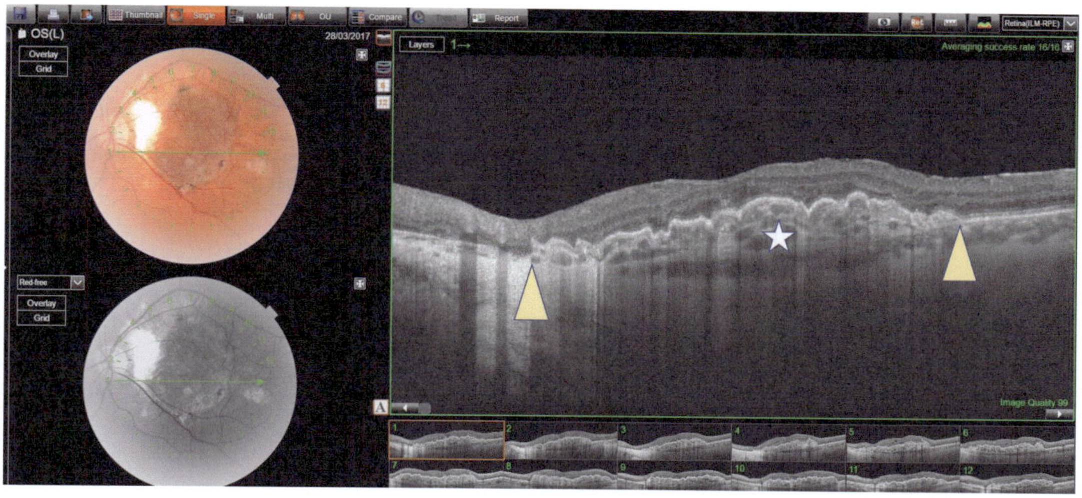

Fig. 9.5 OCT of the patch of choroid and RPE under the retina. The arrowheads delineates the edges of the patch. The retinal layers are well visible. The patch has disomogeneous thickness and dark hyporeflective spaces corresponding to the choroidal vessels (star). The margins of the patch

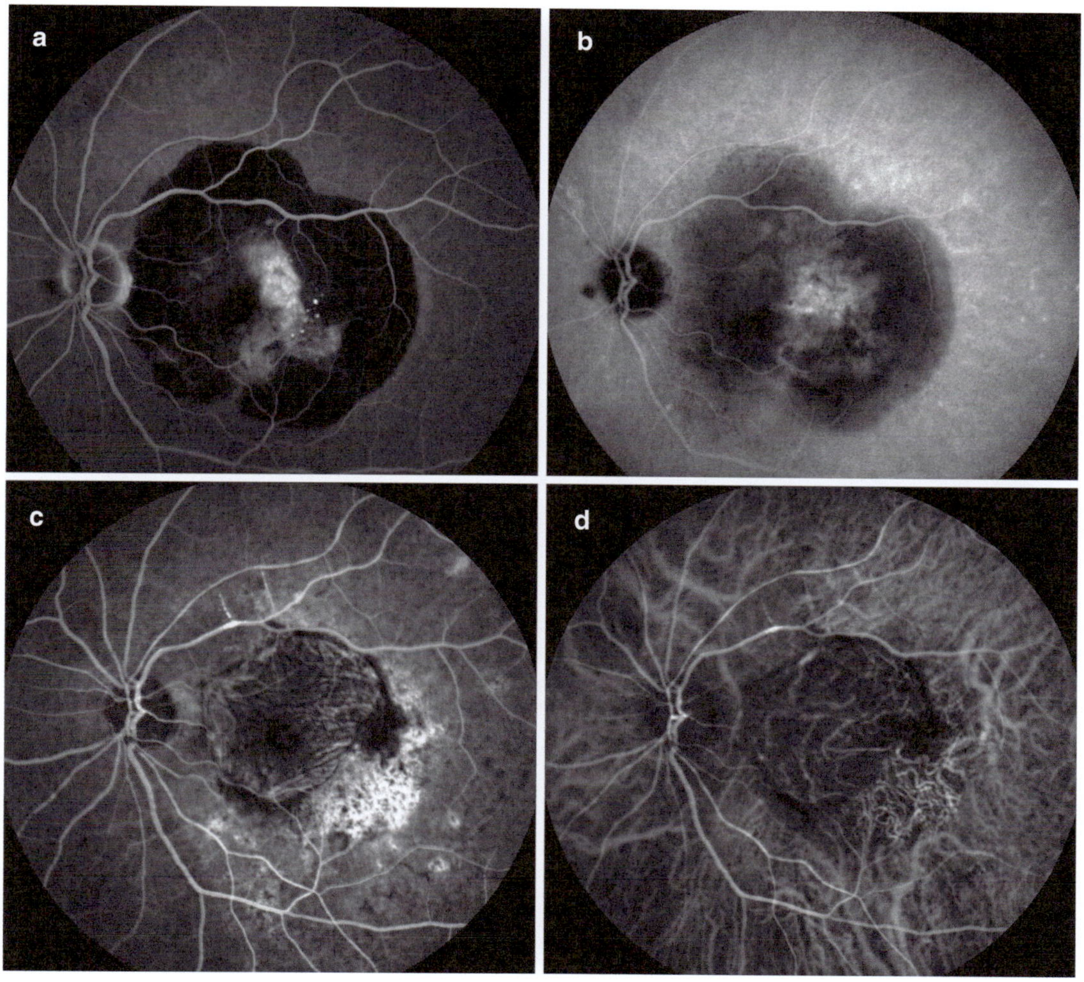

Fig. 9.6 Fluorescein angiography (**a**,**c**) and Indocianine green (**b**,**d**). Preoperatively (**a**,**c**) and one month after surgery (**b**,**d**), respectively confirmed the vascularization of the patch. The choroidal vessels into the patch presented different direction from the vessels of the surrounding choroid

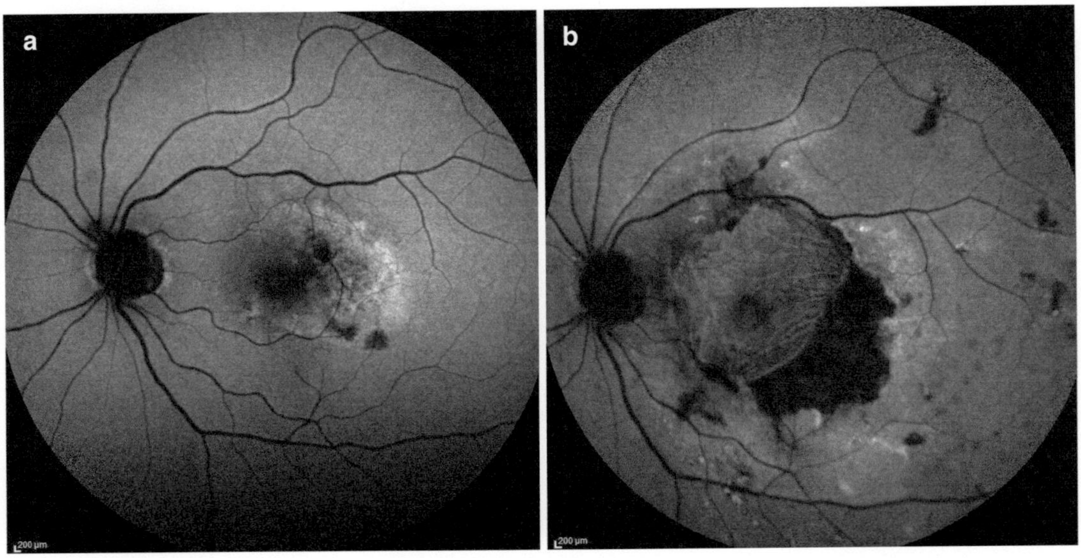

Fig. 9.7 AF preoperatively (**a**) and 1 month after surgery (**b**). AF was normal over the area of the patch and comparable to the AF of the surrounding choroid

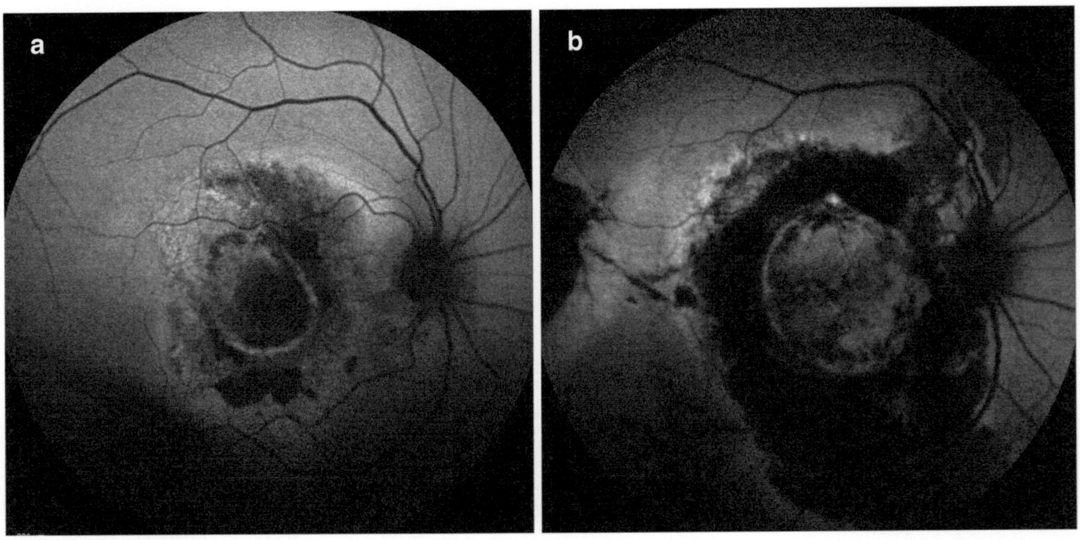

Fig. 9.8 AF preoperatively (**a**) and 6 month after surgery (**b**). Multiple areas of hypoautofluorescence were noticed at the borders of the patch where the necessary surgical manipulation was applied. Some eyes presented scattered areas of hypoautofluorescence also over the patch more than 6 months postoperatively

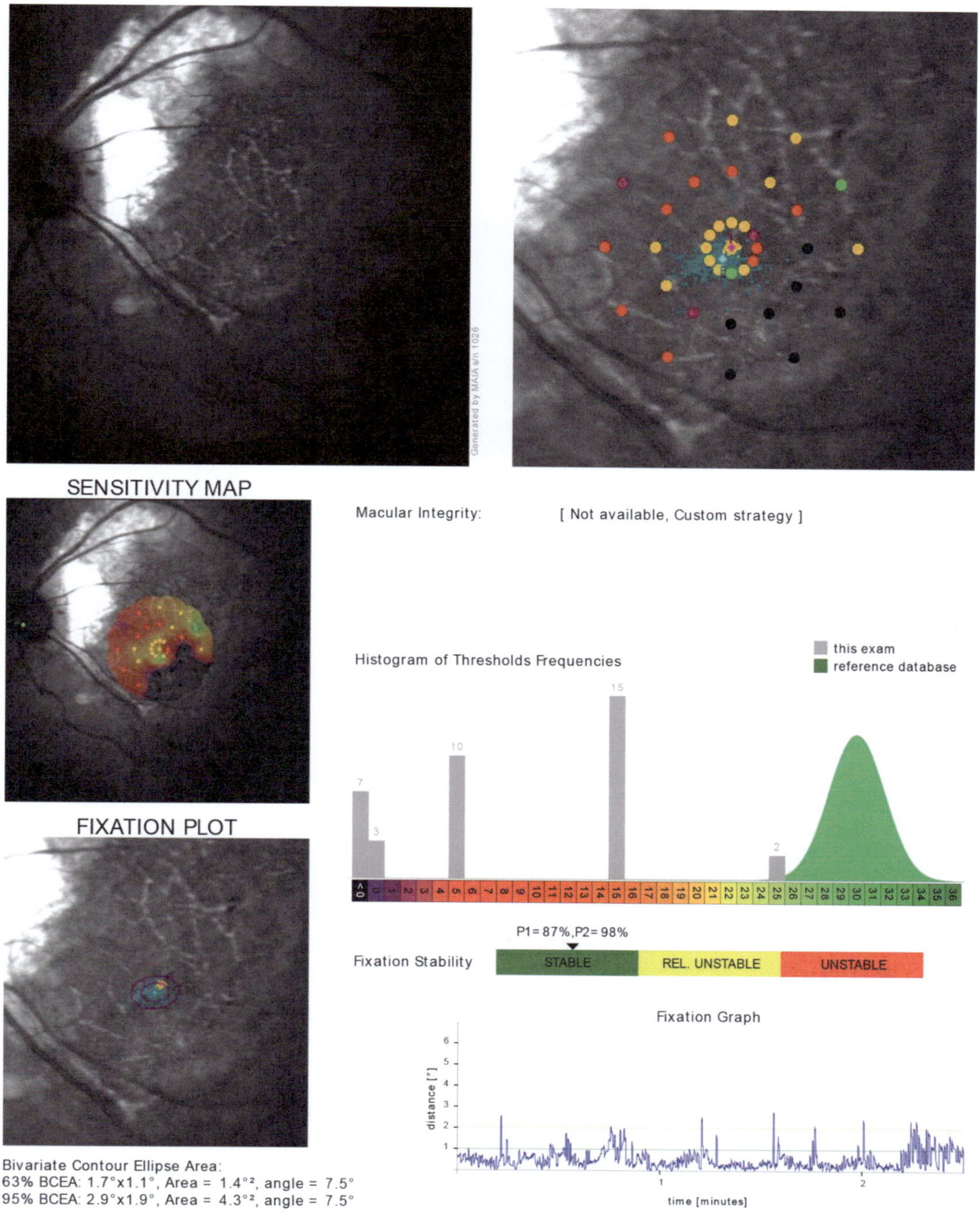

Fig. 9.9 Microperimetry 2 years after surgery showing central fixation and good sensitivity of the retina over more than half of the patch of choroid and RPE

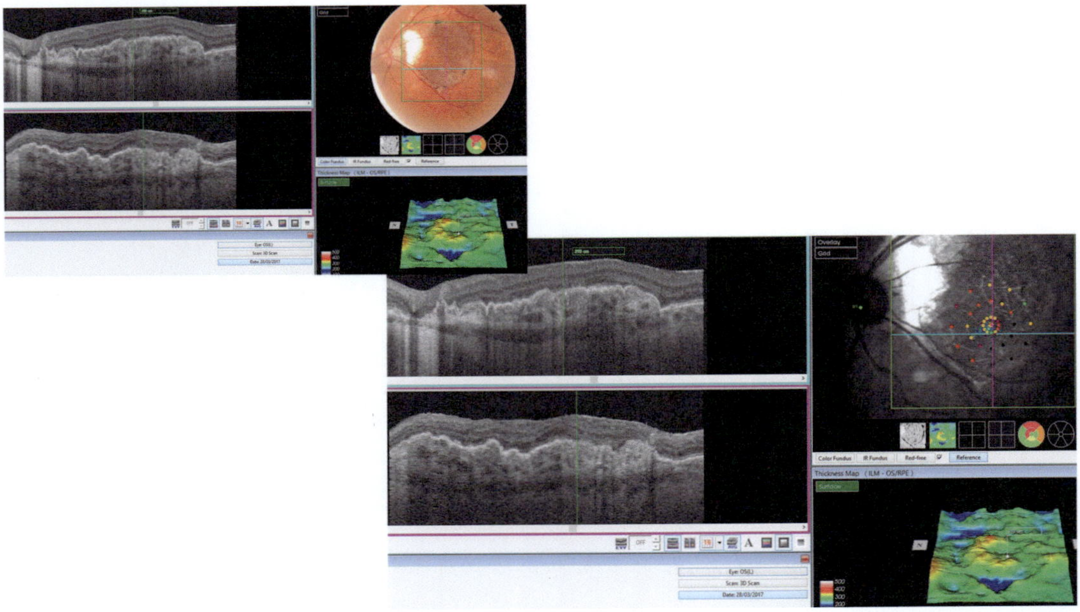

Fig. 9.10 A special software of the OCT Topcon Triton allows to superimpose the OCT image and the microperimetry image to confirm the correspondence of the two exams

References

1. Peyman GA, Blinder KJ, Paris CL, Alturki W, Nelson NC, Desai U. A technique for retinal pigment epithelium transplantation for age-related macular degeneration secondary to extensive subfoveal scarring. Ophthalmic Surg. 1991;22(2):102–8. http://www.ncbi.nlm.nih.gov/pubmed/2038468. Accessed 25 May 2015.
2. Stanga PE, Kychenthal A, Fitzke FW, et al. Retinal pigment epithelium translocation and central visual function in age related macular degeneration: preliminary results. Int Ophthalmol. 2001;23(4–6):297–307. http://www.ncbi.nlm.nih.gov/pubmed/11944854. Accessed 31 May 2015.
3. Van Meurs JC, Van Den Biesen PR. Autologous retinal pigment epithelium and choroid translocation in patients with exudative age-related macular degeneration: short-term follow-up. Am J Ophthalmol. 2003;136(4):688–95. https://doi.org/10.1016/S0002-9394(03)00384-2.
4. Van Meurs JC, ter Averst E, Hofland LJ, et al. Autologous peripheral retinal pigment epithelium translocation in patients with subfoveal neovascular membranes. Br J Ophthalmol. 2004;88(1):110–3. http://www.pubmedcentral.nih.gov/articlerender.fcgi?artid=1771957&tool=pmcentrez&rendertype=abstract. Accessed 31 May 2015.
5. Falkner-Radler CI, Krebs I, Glittenberg C, et al. Human retinal pigment epithelium (RPE) transplantation: outcome after autologous RPE-choroid sheet and RPE cell-suspension in a randomised clinical study. Br J Ophthalmol. 2011;95(3):370–5. https://doi.org/10.1136/bjo.2009.176305.
6. Han L, Ma Z, Wang C, et al. Autologous transplantation of simple retinal pigment epithelium sheet for massive submacular hemorrhage associated with pigment epithelium detachment. Invest Ophthalmol Vis Sci. 2013;54(7):4956–63. https://doi.org/10.1167/iovs.13-11957.
7. Van Zeeburg EJT, Maaijwee KJM, Missotten TOAR, Heimann H, van Meurs JC. A free retinal pigment epithelium-choroid patch in patients with exudative age-related macular degeneration: results up to 7 years. Am J Ophthalmol. 2012;153(1):120–127.e2. https://doi.org/10.1016/j.ajo.2011.06.007.
8. Van Zeeburg EJT, Cereda MG, Amarakoon S, van Meurs JC. Prospective, randomized intervention study comparing retinal pigment epithelium-choroid patch surgery and anti-VEGF therapy in patients with exudative age-related macular degeneration. Ophthalmologica. 2015;233(3–4):134–45. https://doi.org/10.1159/000380829.
9. Cereda MG, Parolini B, Bellesini E, Pertile G. Surgery for CNV and autologous choroidal RPE patch transplantation: exposing the submacular space. Graefes Arch Clin Exp Ophthalmol. 2010;248(1):37–47.
10. Heussen FM, Fawzy NF, Joeres S, et al. Autologous translocation of the choroid and RPE in age-related macular degeneration: 1-year follow-up in 30 patients and recommendations for patient selection. Eye (Lond). 2008;22(6):799–807. https://doi.org/10.1038/sj.eye.6702823.
11. Joussen AM, Heussen FM, Joeres S, et al. Autologous translocation of the choroid and retinal pigment epithelium in age-related macular degeneration. Am J Ophthalmol. 2006;142(1):17–30. https://doi.org/10.1016/j.ajo.2006.01.090.

Index

L.-O. Hattenbach (ed.), *Management of Macular Hemorrhage*,
https://doi.org/10.1007/978-3-319-65877-3

MIX
Papier aus verantwortungsvollen Quellen
Paper from responsible sources
FSC® C105338

If you have any concerns about our products,
you can contact us on
ProductSafety@springernature.com

In case Publisher is established outside the EU,
the EU authorized representative is:
Springer Nature Customer Service Center GmbH
Europaplatz 3, 69115 Heidelberg, Germany

Printed by Libri Plureos GmbH
in Hamburg, Germany